Clinical Microbiology
Quality in Laboratory Diagnosis

Diagnostic Standards of Care

MICHAEL LAPOSATA, MD, PHD
Series Editor

Coagulation Disorders
Quality in Laboratory Diagnosis
Michael Laposata, MD, PhD

Clinical Microbiology
Quality in Laboratory Diagnosis
Charles W. Stratton, MD

Forthcoming in the Series
Laboratory Management
Clinical Chemistry
Transfusion Medicine
Hematology / Immunology

Diagnostic Standards of Care Series

Clinical Microbiology
Quality in Laboratory Diagnosis

Charles W. Stratton, MD

Associate Professor of Pathology and Medicine
Department of Pathology
Vanderbilt University School of Medicine
Director, Clinical Microbiology Laboratory
Vanderbilt University Hospital
Nashville, Tennessee

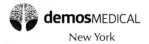
demosMEDICAL
New York

Visit our website at www.demosmedpub.com

ISBN: 978-1-936287-19-2
E-book ISBN: 978-1-6170-5048-0

Acquisitions Editor: Richard Winters
Compositor: S4Carlisle Publishing Services
Printer: Gasch Printing

Medicine is an ever-changing science. Research and clinical experience are continually expanding our knowledge, in particular our understanding of proper treatment and drug therapy. The authors, editors, and publisher have made every effort to ensure that all information in this book is in accordance with the state of knowledge at the time of production of the book. Nevertheless, the authors, editors, and publisher are not responsible for errors or omissions or for any consequences from application of the information in this book and make no warranty, express or implied, with respect to the contents of the publication. Every reader should examine carefully the package inserts accompanying each drug and should carefully check whether the dosage schedules mentioned therein or the contraindications stated by the manufacturer differ from the statements made in this book. Such examination is particularly important with drugs that are either rarely used or have been newly released on the market.

Library of Congress Cataloging-in-Publication Data
Stratton, Charles W.
    Clinical microbiology : quality in laboratory diagnosis / Charles W. Stratton.
        p.; cm.—(Diagnostic standards of care series)
Includes bibliographical references and index.
    ISBN 978-1-936287-19-2 (alk. paper)
    1. Medical microbiology. 2. Diagnostic microbiology—Quality control. I. Title.
    II. Series: Diagnostic standards of care.
    [DNLM: 1. Microbiological Techniques—methods. 2. Diagnostic Errors—prevention & control. 3. Laboratory Techniques and Procedures—standards. 4. Quality Control. QW 25]
    QR46.S863 2011
    616.9'041—dc23

                                                                      2011021516

Made in the United States of America
11 12 13 14/ 5 4 3 2 1

To my wife, Pia, who is the "Wind in My Sails."

Contents

Series Foreword

"Above all, do no harm." This frequently quoted admonition to healthcare providers is highly regarded, but despite that, there are few books, if any, that focus primarily on how to avoid harming patients by learning from the mistakes of others.

Would it not be of great benefit to patients if all healthcare providers were aware of the thrombotic consequences from heparin induced thrombocytopenia before a patient's leg is amputated? The clinically significant, often lethal, thrombotic events that occur in patients who develop heparin induced thrombocytopenia would be greatly diminished if all healthcare providers appropriately monitored platelet counts in patients being treated with intravenous unfractionated heparin.

It was a desire to learn from the mistakes of others that led to the concept for this series of books on diagnostic standards of care. As the test menu in the clinical laboratory has enlarged in size and complexity, errors in selection of tests and errors in the interpretation of test results have become commonplace, and these mistakes can result in poor patient outcomes. This series of books on diagnostic standards of care in coagulation, microbiology, transfusion medicine, hematology, clinical chemistry, immunology, and laboratory management are all organized in a similar fashion. Clinical errors, and accompanying cases to illustrate each error, are presented within all of the chapters in several discrete categories: errors in test selection, errors in result interpretation, other errors, and diagnostic controversies. Each chapter concludes with a summary list of the standards of care. The most common errors made by thousands of healthcare providers daily are the ones that have been selected for presentation in this series of books.

Practicing physicians ordering tests with which they are less familiar would benefit significantly by learning of the potential errors associated with ordering such tests and errors associated with interpreting an infrequently encountered test result. Medical trainees who are gaining clinical experience would benefit significantly by first understanding what not to do when it comes to ordering laboratory tests and interpreting test results from the clinical laboratory. Individuals working in the clinical laboratory would also benefit by learning of the common mistakes made by healthcare providers so that they are better able to provide helpful advice that would avert the damaging consequences of an error. Finally, laboratory managers and hospital administrators would benefit by having knowledge of test ordering mistakes to improve the efficiency of the clinical laboratory and avoid the cost of performing unnecessary tests.

If the errors described in this series of books could be greatly reduced, the savings to the healthcare system and the improvement in patient outcomes would be dramatic.

Michael Laposata, MD, PhD
Series Editor

Preface

It is the purpose of this book to address common medical errors seen in the clinical microbiology laboratory, to allow these errors to be appreciated by both clinicians and laboratorians. The errors will be addressed using the following phases of testing; preanalytic testing phase, analytic testing phase, and postanalytic testing phase. In particular, those medical errors in the preanalytic and postanalytic testing phases will be stressed, as errors in the analytic phase of testing have been addressed for a much longer period of time by quality assurance (QA) programs [1,2] that ensure that the information generated by the clinical microbiology laboratory is accurate, reliable, and reproducible. Finally, the medical errors will be described and discussed in a clinical case-based learning format to effectively illustrate the conditions that contribute to these errors. Clinical cases will include those published in the medical literature as well as those observed by the author. Those medical errors that are more common and/or more important will be illustrated with a larger number of cases than those that are less common.

Medical errors in the clinical microbiology laboratory can be divided into three phases: preanalytic, analytic, and postanalytic. In clinical microbiology, the preanalytic phase involves selecting and ordering the test, collecting the specimen, and transporting the specimen to the laboratory. This preanalytic phase is extremely important, as a mistake here may result in failure to identify the microorganism that is causing the infection. For example, meningococci in CSF perish if not rapidly cultured; a false-negative result of a CSF culture that was delayed in terms of being cultured by the clinical microbiology laboratory could be life threatening [3]. The analytic phase is the actual testing that occurs in the clinical microbiology laboratory. An example of a medical error that might occur in the analytic phase would be a medical technologist misreading a Gram stain. Such internal problems and errors are well recognized within the clinical microbiology laboratory [1,2,4]; this recognition has led to both internal [1] and external [2] quality assessment programs. Moreover, laboratorians, government agencies, and suppliers have worked together to create voluntary consensus standards [5,6]. This work, in part, has resulted in the formation of the National Committee for Clinical Laboratory Standards (NCCLS), which has been renamed Clinical Laboratory Standards Institute (CLSI). The published standards/guidelines from NCCLS/CLSI have provided the basis for uniform testing procedures in the clinical microbiology laboratory [6]. As a result, medical errors occurring within the clinical microbiology laboratory have been greatly reduced. The postanalytic phase includes both reporting the laboratory result to the clinician and the clinician's interpretation of that result. For example, the clinical microbiology laboratory may report isolation of *Streptococcus anginosus* from a blood culture, but it is the clinician's interpretation of this result as likely pointing toward a deep-seated source of underlying infection that required a thorough diagnostic evaluation that is the critical factor for this particular infected patient [7]. Each of the steps in these three phases can have an adverse impact on the diagnosis and treatment of an infectious disease if a medical error occurs.

Charles W. Stratton, MD

Preanalytic Errors in the Clinical Microbiology Laboratory

OVERVIEW

Clinical microbiologists are well aware of the adage first coined by computer programmers, "garbage in, garbage out," but for their profession have renamed it "quality in, quality out." Their adage refers to the fact that the quality of the clinical specimen received by the clinical microbiology laboratory is a key factor in the optimal use of clinical microbiology. For serological testing, the timing of the serum collection may be an equally critical factor for optimal use. Unfortunately, the clinicians often do not have the tools, interest, training, access to data, or time to determine optimal use of the clinical microbiology laboratory for their patients.

The clinical case reports in this chapter are selected from the medical literature and the personal experiences of the author. They illustrate common preanalytic medical errors in the clinical microbiology laboratory.

FAILURE TO CONSIDER INFECTION

> ▶ Failure to consider infection is actually a more common problem than one might think. It seems to center around surgical procedures where a malignancy is suspected. Thus, oncologists and surgeons must be alert and always consider the possibility of infection even when malignancy is their first concern.

Case with Averted Error

A previously healthy 5-month-old girl was seen at a hospital located in the southeastern United States; this infant presented with a 1-week history of fever and irritability. The infant's physical examination was notable for a distended abdomen with a liver edge palpable 5 cm below the right costal margin and a spleen tip palpable 3 to 4 cm below the left costal margin. Initial laboratory findings included a complete blood count with a white blood cell count of 6,180/μL, a hemoglobin level of 8.6 g/dL, and a platelet count of 96,000/μL. No blasts were seen on the peripheral blood smears. Bacterial cultures of blood, urine, and cerebrospinal fluid were obtained. The infant was admitted to the hospital and received empirical antimicrobial therapy. Following admission, a pediatric hematology/oncology consultant evaluated the infant due to the fever, hepatosplenomegaly, and pancytopenia. The hematology/oncology consultant noted that all of the bacterial cultures were negative. In the presence of fever and hepatosplenomegaly with leucopenia, thrombocytopenia, and anemia, regardless of whether blasts are noted on the peripheral blood smears, the hematology/oncology consultant was particularly concerned with malignancy. In this age group, the most common malignant disorders with these presenting symptoms and signs include acute and chronic lymphoblastic leukemia and lymphomas. Fever may be a symptom in the initial presentation of such patients. Therefore, the pediatric hematology/oncology consultant recommended bone marrow aspiration and biopsy, which was done. The bone marrow aspiration and biopsy showed no evidence of a hematologic malignancy. At this point, the possibility of infection was raised. Specifically, disseminated histoplasmosis was considered as this patient lived in the southeastern United States. Unfortunately, fungal cultures (or any cultures at all) had not been ordered on the bone marrow aspirate and biopsy, as infection had not been considered when this test was ordered. Hematoxylin and eosin (H&E) and special stains on the bone marrow biopsy were done and revealed noncaseating granulomas without fungal organisms. Based on these histological findings, serum and urine *Histoplasma* antigen tests [8] were ordered. Both the serum and the urine *Histoplasma* antigen tests were positive, and a diagnosis of disseminated histoplasmosis was made. Disseminated histoplasmosis of infancy often presents with a characteristic triad of fever, hepatosplenomegaly, and hematologic abnormalities [9]. Infants with disseminated histoplasmosis are frequently referred to hematologists or oncologists to rule out leukemia or lymphoma as the underlying cause of their symptoms/signs. Often the diagnosis is only suspected after the peripheral blood smear and bone marrow biopsy specimen has failed to demonstrate a malignancy. If fungal cultures are not ordered on the bone marrow biopsy, an opportunity to diagnose disseminated histoplasmosis may be lost. Fortunately, the availability of serum and urine *Histoplasma* antigen tests allowed this infant to be successfully diagnosed and treated for disseminated histoplasmosis.

Explanation and Consequences

Failure to consider an infection is an obvious situation where not sending material from a clinical specimen to the clinical microbiology laboratory for culture or other microbiological testing may result in a preanalytic medical error. This is a very subtle type of medical error and is considered an individual type of error that is not easily rectified by a systems approach. As illustrated by this case, the situation may occur when the initial clinical impression suggests malignancy. Bone marrow aspirations and biopsies are often done to rule out malignancy; cultures may not be requested on the aspirate/biopsy as the clinicians are focused on malignancy and not thinking about infection. In this case, the error was averted by the availability of the *Histoplasma* antigen test, which allowed the diagnosis to be made.

Case with Error

This case [10] involves a 30-year-old man who presented with a chief complaint of severe pain in the lumbar spine followed by pain in the cervical spine with restriction in the range of movement of his head. Of note is that 18 years earlier this patient had been successfully treated for acute lymphatic T-cell leukemia (T-ALL) with polychemotherapy and irradiation of the skull. Because of this history of T-ALL, a recurrence was suspected. Therefore, the patient was referred to hematology/oncology consultants who directed the initial evaluation of this lumbar and cervical pain. A tine test for tuberculosis at this time was noted to be positive. A computed tomography scan revealed osteolytic lesions in the spine, pelvis, and ribs; a bone marrow biopsy of the right iliac crest was done to rule out recurrence of T-cell lymphoma. Although this biopsy did not reveal bone marrow malignancy, a diagnosis of acute lymphatic leukemia with bone involvement was made and induction chemotherapy was initiated. The patient's bone pain increased and the osteolytic lesions progressed and eventually involved the perivertebral tissues. In addition, an abscess had developed at the puncture site of the right iliac crest. Material from this abscess was cultured and was sterile; an acid-fast stain of this material was negative. At this time, laboratory values included a white blood cell count of 12,000/µL and an elevated C-reactive protein. A diagnosis of tuberculosis was considered, and the patient empirically received a short course of antituberculosis therapy with rifampin, isoniazid, and pyrazinamide. Doubt was cast on the correctness of the diagnosis of tuberculosis due to the absence of positive cultures for *Mycobacterium tuberculosis* as well as the absence of acid-fast bacilli. Instead, a diagnosis of chronic recurrent multifocal osteomyelitis was made, and antituberculosis therapy was stopped. Treatment with high-dose prednisone and indomethacin was initiated with marked improvement of the patient's symptoms. Attempts to reduce the steroid dose were unsuccessful as symptoms recurred. Ultimately, the patient complained of right-sided abdominal pain; a computed tomography scan revealed an extensive abscess involving the liver and lesser pelvis. Surgical treatment of the abscess resulted in material that was acid-fast positive and grew *M. avium-intracellulare*.

A quadruple combination of rifampin, isoniazid, clarithromycin, and ethambutol was initiated and led to complete resolution of the osteolytic lesions after 2 years of treatment.

Explanation and Consequences

This is another case in which the failure to consider infection was a medical error and may have delayed the diagnosis and treatment of a *M. avium-intracellulare* infection of the bone. Cultures of the initial bone marrow biopsy from the iliac crest were not done and would have been more likely to be positive than were the cultures of the abscess material that were done at a later time. *M. avium-intracellulare* is known to disseminate [11] and can involve the bone [12]. In this patient, the previous history of acute lymphatic leukemia led to the incorrect conclusion that these osteolytic lesions were due to recurrent ALL despite the fact that the medical literature reports no case of ALL that exclusively involved the bones [10]. The diagnosis of chronic recurrent multifocal osteomyelitis [12] seemed plausible in a scenario of seemingly sterile osteomyelitis. However, the bone marrow biopsy of the right ileac crest was not cultured although the abscess material was cultured. Therefore, this did not truly represent sterile osteomyelitis. Moreover, extension of osteolytic lesions into adjacent tissue with formation of abscesses is not typically seen in chronic recurrent multifocal osteomyelitis [13]. Had the clinicians considered infection as a possible cause of multiple osteolytic lesions and done appropriate cultures (i.e., routine, fungal, and mycobacterial cultures) on the initial bone marrow biopsy, the diagnosis of nontuberculous osteomyelitis might have been made earlier.

Case with Error

This case [14] involves a 54-year-old woman who presented with a chief complaint of a gradually enlarging right submandibular mass of several months' duration. Her past medical history was remarkable only for well-controlled hypothyroidism. She had been treated with two courses of oral cephalexin with no improvement. She was otherwise asymptomatic. When an adult patient presents with a neck mass, malignancy is the greatest concern with fine-needle aspiration and biopsy being one of the best techniques for evaluating such a neck mass [15]. Indeed, it has been recommended that an excisional biopsy be obtained when a neck mass persists beyond 4 to 6 weeks after a single course of a broad-spectrum antibiotic [15]. Therefore, this patient received a fine-needle aspiration that was nondiagnostic. Cultures of the aspiration were not done. The patient subsequently developed a draining fistula tract. At this point, excision of the mass was appropriately done for diagnostic purposes, and a necrotic mass was found next to the right submandibular gland. Further excision of the fistulous tract, right submandibular gland, and surrounding lymph nodes was done. On histopathological examination, two of the five excised lymph nodes and the fistula tract exhibited necrotizing granulomatous inflammation. Gram stains, Gomori-methenamine silver stains, and acid-fast stains were all negative for microorganisms. Fortunately, material from these lymph nodes had been sent for appropriate cultures including those for mycobacteria; at 2 weeks the mycobacterial culture became positive with an acid-fast bacterium. This bacterium was identified as *M. avium* complex. As the patient's incision from the biopsy had healed well and a follow-up computed tomography scan noted no additional masses, no antituberculosis therapy was done [16]. The patient did well and had no recurrence of this neck mass at 6 months.

Explanation and Consequences

In this case, a malignancy was a valid concern, which led to a fine-needle aspiration and biopsy. This concern and diagnostic approach is appropriate. However, had this aspiration/biopsy been cultured, a diagnosis might have been made sooner although the subsequent draining fistula would still have required excision of the neck mass and fistula tract. Had the excised lymph nodes and sinus tract not been cultured, this diagnosis might have been missed. Failure to consider infection can be seen in a patient with neck mass and/or cervical lymphadenopathy [17] in which lymphoma [18] or metastatic carcinoma [19] is the working diagnosis. Because lymph node biopsy is often reserved for situations in which a malignant process is suspected, the clinician may not think to order cultures [20–22]. For example, a biopsy for asymptomatic cervical lymphadenopathy of greater than 3 weeks' duration is a common situation in which metastatic carcinoma is suspected, particularly in patients over 40 years of age [23,24]—exactly the clinical situation seen in this illustrative case. These enlarged cervical lymph nodes thus are usually excised or biopsied, and the lymphatic tissue is sent to the surgical pathology laboratory. If cultures are desired, the surgeon must send part of the lymphatic tissue to the clinical microbiology laboratory. Lymphatic tissue sent to the surgical pathology laboratory is fixed in formalin, which precludes additional tests such as tissue cultures when the H&E examination reveals lymphadenitis [20–23]. Failure to send part of the lymphatic tissue to the clinical microbiology laboratory for culture is a particular problem in children where nontuberculous cervical lymphadenopathy is more commonly seen [21,22,25]. Infections that may present with cervical lymphadenopathy include cervical mycobacterial infections [21,22,25,26] (*M. tuberculosis* and *M. avian* complex), cat scratch disease (*Bartonella henselae*) [27,28], histoplasmosis [29,30], and toxoplasmosis [31,32].

Case with Error

This case [33] is that of a 7-month-old infant who was referred to a pediatric hospital because of a 4-month history of breathlessness not associated with fever, cachexia, or night sweats. The patient's symptoms had not been responsive to a course of antimicrobial therapy for possible pneumonia. There was no history suggestive of foreign-body ingestion. On physical examination, the infant was noted to have decreased breath sounds at the base of the right chest; no lymphadenopathy was noted. A plain chest radiograph demonstrated a perihilar mass on the right side; this mass had caused a mediastinal shift and collapse of the right lower lobe. This perihilar mass was suspicious of a mediastinal tumor. Indeed, the most common causes of mediastinal masses in children are tumors [34]. A computed tomography scan demonstrated a large superior mediastinal mass extending inferiorly into the right hemithorax; irregular areas of calcification and the absence of cavities gave this mass the appearance of a neuroblastoma. Blood and urinary catecholamines, and serum beta-HCG were normal;

alpha-fetoprotein and LDH were noted to be mildly elevated. A thoracoscopy was done and confirmed the mass and also demonstrated multiple pleural seedlings; the mass and pleural seedlings were biopsied. No tissue was sent to the clinical microbiology laboratory for microbial cultures, as tumor was the suspected diagnosis. However, histopathologic evaluation of this tissue and pleural seedlings revealed a diagnosis of tuberculosis. The infant was treated for tuberculosis and recovered. An epidemiologic evaluation identified a tuberculosis contact in the family's shared accommodation.

Explanation and Consequences

Biopsy of indeterminate mediastinal masses is often done in order to evaluate the mediastinal mass/lymph nodes for malignancy [34–38]. As illustrated by this case, tissue may not be sent to the clinical microbiology laboratory for cultures, as malignancy is the considered the most likely cause of the mediastinal mass. When histopathologic examination reveals no malignancy, the opportunity for culture has passed. The demonstration of microorganisms by special stains may provide the diagnosis, as it did in this case. Tuberculosis is an unusual cause of mediastinal mass in an infant, and such cases have rarely been reported [33,39]. In contrast, histoplasmosis as a cause of mediastinal mass in an infant or in a child has been reported on many occasions [40–42]. Of importance is that often these cases of mediastinal histoplasmosis in children were mistakenly diagnosed as lymphoma [40,41]. In one series of 37 children with mediastinal mass, 16 had biopsy-proved lymphoma while 21 had histoplasmosis [41]. Clearly there is a significant risk for medical errors in cases involving a mediastinal mass in a child if infection is not considered.

Case with Error

This case [43] involves a 35-year-old woman, gravida 1, para 1, who was referred to a tertiary care medical center from another hospital for evaluation of a suspected ovarian cancer for which she had received operative treatment 3 weeks previously. The patient had complained of abdominal pain, increasing abdominal girth, adnexal masses, diarrhea, fever, and weight loss over the preceding 4 months. Moreover, a diagnosis of hydronephrosis of the right kidney had been made at the outside hospital. An intrauterine device (IUD) had been placed 9 years previously, but had been removed 2 months before admission to the outside hospital. The patient's past medical history was otherwise unremarkable. At the outside hospital, an exploratory laparotomy had been performed; biopsies of the peritoneum showed no evidence of malignancy. Despite the negative biopsies, diffuse peritoneal carcinomatosis was suspected. The patient received a right nephrostomy and was referred for further treatment of the presumed ovarian carcinoma. The physical examination at the referral hospital revealed a fixed pelvic mass extending to both pelvic walls and to the posterior sacral region. Assessment of the lower abdomen by transvaginal and transabdominal sonography revealed solid hypoechogenic-appearing adnexal masses with cystic components and without blood flow. Normal ovaries were not detected. Ascites was not detected. Laboratory values included a white blood cell count of 11,900/μL, a hemoglobin of 9.8 g/dL, an elevated C-reactive protein, and a slightly elevated C-125 tumor marker. A diagnostic laparotomy was performed and revealed intestinal adhesions and bilateral tubo-ovarian abscesses; all pelvic structures were covered with marked fibrosis. A bilateral salpingo-oophorectomy was performed and drainage of the pelvic region was established. The histopathologic examination of the ovaries and fallopian tubes revealed no evidence of malignancy, but sulfur granules were noted. These sulfur granules led to the diagnosis of extensive actinomycosis of both ovaries and fallopian tubes. Antimicrobial therapy was initiated with ampicillin/sulbactam; this resulted in compete resolution of the induration and masses in the pelvis after 2 weeks of therapy. The patient has remained well without any symptoms for 2 years following her surgery.

Explanation and Consequences

This case illustrates another situation in which failure to consider infection can lead to a medical error. The incidence of IUD-associated cervicovaginal actinomycosis has been shown to be between 8% and 16% in several studies [44,45]. Actinomycotic pelvic inflammatory disease resulting from IUD-associated cervicovaginal actinomycosis is a well-described mimic of ovarian cancer [43,46–49]. For example, Fiorino reviewed the medical literature in 1996 and found 92 cases in 63 reports describing actinomycotic pelvic inflammatory disease mimicking ovarian cancer [47]. A number of cases of ovarian actinomycosis mimicking malignancy in which there was no IUD involved also have been described [48]. Clearly, actinomycosis should be included in the differential diagnosis of pelvic masses, especially in patients with a history of IUD use. Surgical exploration of a pelvic mass should include appropriate biopsy specimens sent to the clinical microbiology laboratory for Gram stain and anaerobic cultures as well as biopsy specimens sent to the surgical pathology laboratory for histopathologic evaluation. It should be noted that actinomycosis mimics malignancy in other tissues as well, including tonsillar tissue [50], pancreas [51], intestine [52–54], liver [55,56], and kidney [57].

Case with Averted Error

This case [58] involves a 70-year-old male from Arizona who was referred to a medical center in Tennessee as a potential candidate for robotically assisted radical prostatectomy. His past medical history was significant for prostate cancer as well as a 2-year history of cough that had been previously diagnosed in Arizona as new onset asthma. The patient was afebrile and had an unremarkable physical examination except for previously noted enlargement of his prostate. A macrocytic anemia and an eosinophila of 16.5% were noted on his complete blood count; laboratory values were otherwise unremarkable. A computed tomography scan was done as part of his initial evaluation in order to exclude the metastatic spread of prostate cancer; this scan revealed multiple, bilateral pulmonary nodules. The pulmonary nodules ranged in size from 1–2 mm to 9 mm and were accompanied by bulky mediastinal and hilar lymphadenopathy. These pulmonary nodules and mediastinal/hilar lymphadenopathy were thought to represent metastatic spread of the prostate cancer. A bronchoscopy with fine-needle aspiration of the pulmonary nodules plus a paratracheal lymph node was done to confirm the presumed diagnosis of malignancy. However, in this case, a potential medical error was avoided as the presence of the peripheral eosinophilia in a patient from Arizona alerted a pathologist to the possibility of coccidioidomycosis [59]. Therefore, cultures were done on material obtained by fine-needle aspiration. Histopathologic examination of material obtained by fine-needle aspiration was unremarkable; cultures grew *Coccidioides immitis*. Without these cultures, an additional surgical procedure might have been needed to make this diagnosis. The patient was treated with fluconazole and had marked symptomatic improvement; an uncomplicated prostatectomy was also successfully done.

Explanation and Consequences

Lung infections mimicking malignancy are well described in the medical literature [60–65]. An important reason for this is that both pulmonary infections and pulmonary malignancies are initially detected by a radiologic diagnostic procedure such as a chest radiograph x-ray or a chest computed tomography scan. Radiologic features suggestive of a pulmonary malignancy include a parenchymal mass with speculated margins, microlobulations, thick-walled cavity, cavity showing nodular margins, and chest wall invasion [64]. These findings, however, are not specific and can be seen with pulmonary infections. If the possibility of an infection is not considered, the diagnostic procedures done may not include those measures such as culture that are necessary to detect infection. In this illustrative case, histopathologic examination of the fine-needle aspiration specimen were unrevealing while the culture of this material provided the diagnosis of coccidioidomycosis. This case is similar to other cases reported in the medical literature. For example, in one large series of over 2,000 patients who underwent a lung biopsy with a presumed diagnosis of malignancy, 37 (1.3%) of these cases were found to have infection rather than malignancy [60]. Fungal infections accounted for 46% of the infections diagnosed in this series. Clearly the possibility of infection must be kept in mind when initiating diagnostic procedures to confirm a presumed pulmonary malignancy.

STANDARDS OF CARE

■ Failure to consider infection can result in a medical error when material from biopsy specimens is not sent to the clinical microbiology laboratory because malignancy is considered the most likely diagnosis; when the tissue turns out to not be malignant, the lack of a culture result may result in harm to the patient.

■ Conversely, sending material for culture from a tissue biopsy specimen that ultimately turns out to be malignant is not considered a medical error; the culture will not grow and no harm to the patient will result.

■ Oncologists and surgeons, in particular, must remember that infections are able to mimic malignancy; therefore, obtaining cultures of biopsy tissues should be carefully considered when biopsies are being done to rule out or confirm suspected cancer.

FAILURE TO CONSIDER UNCOMMON INFECTIONS

> ▶ Failure to consider uncommon infections is another common medical error seen in infectious diseases and clinical microbiology. This type of error is best avoided by obtaining consultation (informal or formal) from infectious disease clinicians and/or the clinical microbiology laboratory director.

Case with Error

This case [66] involves a 73-year-old man who was admitted to the hospital in early summer with a chief complaint of fever, weakness, and pain in the muscles of his legs. The patient had been well until 1 week before admission, when he had the onset of a dry cough and rhinorrhea lasting 2 days. Three weeks prior to admission, the patient had traveled to Cape Cod, Massachusetts. Six days prior to admission, the patient had traveled from Boston to coastal South Carolina to attend a conference. There was no history of tick bites during either of these trips. Three months prior to admission, the patient had been started on atorvastatin for the treatment of an elevated cholesterol level. The past medical history was otherwise noncontributory. Three days prior to admission, the patient had experienced severe myalgias in both thighs as well as a temperature as high as 39.4°C. He elected to treat himself with bed rest because he thought he had the "flu." The patient next experienced generalized weakness and extension of his myalgias to include both calf and thigh muscles. The patient at this time also noted increased urinary frequency and one episode of urinary incontinence. The patient continued to think he had the "flu" and therefore remained in bed. However, the patient's wife brought him to the emergency room as his fever was continuing and he was feeling worse. On physical examination, the patient appeared acutely ill and was unsteady on his feet; vital signs included a temperature of 39°C, a pulse of 84 bpm, and a B/P of 145/80 mm Hg. A grade 2 systolic ejection murmur was heard at the left sternal border; the patient had no previous history of cardiac murmurs. The prostate was found to be slightly enlarged and nontender. The remainder of the physical examination was noncontributory. Initial laboratory values included a white blood cell count of 5,800/μL with a left shift, a platelet count of 79,000/μL, and mildly elevated liver function studies. A creatine kinase was noted to be 3,468 IU/L. The urine analysis revealed 3 to 5 RBCs per high-power field and 5 to 10 WBCs per high-power field; many bacteria were noted. The patient was admitted with an initial concern of urosepsis and/or prostatitis even though the prostate was not tender. Blood and urine cultures were obtained, and treatment with trimethoprim-sulfamethoxazole and gentamicin was initiated. On the second day of hospitalization, the patient's temperature again rose to 39°C. His white blood cell count had decreased to 4,000/μL with leucopenia noted, while the platelet count had dropped to 41,000/μL; the blood and urine cultures were no growth at this time. The creatine kinase had increased to 4,833 IU/L. The lack of response to antimicrobial therapy combined with negative blood and urine cultures after 24 hours made the initial concerns of urosepsis appear less likely. Moreover, the white blood cell count did not support the diagnosis of urosepsis. The empirical antimicrobial therapy was changed to ampicillin, levofloxacin, and metronidazole, and an infectious diseases consultation was obtained. Other possible infectious etiologies were considered. In particular, the clinical picture of a severe influenza-like illness occurring in the summertime (so-called "summer flu" [67]) combined with the leucopenia and thrombocytopenia suggested a diagnosis of ehrlichiosis [66–69]; a course of doxycycline was initiated and resulted in clinical resolution of this infection. A PCR assay [70] confirmed this diagnosis, and the patient recovered from this illness. A serologic test done several weeks later also was positive for ehrlichiosis at >1:64 IgG.

Explanation and Consequences

The failure of a clinician to consider an uncommon infection such as ehrlichiosis/anaplasmosis in the differential diagnosis of a febrile patient with "summer flu" [67] may, at best, delay the diagnosis of this infection. At worse, a delay in the diagnosis of ehrlichiosis may result in death [69,71]. A failure to consider the diagnosis of ehrlichiosis in a timely manner may represent an individual failure (failure to consider this infection) or a systems failure (failure of the clinical microbiology laboratory to have a PCR test available for the diagnosis of ehrlichiosis/ anaplasmosis). In this case, the clinicians initially taking care of this patient were concerned with urosepsis, but realized the need to consider other possibilities by the second day of hospitalization and thus consulted an infectious diseases clinician. At this time, the diagnosis of ehrlichiosis was considered, given the clinical picture of fever, leucopenia, and thrombocytopenia as well as the history of travel to South Carolina. Accordingly, empirical therapy with doxycycline was started, and the appropriate PCR assay was obtained. Ehrlichiosis can cause significant morbidity and mortality if not suspected and treated promptly [69,71]. Recognition of ehrlichiosis/anaplasmosis as a possible diagnosis in this type of clinical situation clearly requires the treating clinician to have knowledge about such tickborne illnesses, which are an emerging infectious threat [72,73]. Alternatively, consultation with an infectious diseases clinician may avoid such a medical error. Serologic testing does not usually help in the diagnosis of acute ehrlichiosis, as seroconversion may not occur until 3 weeks into the illness [66–68]. Treatment thus should be initiated based on the clinical presentation and not based on the results of laboratory testing. A PCR assay for ehrlichiosis is an alternative method for diagnosing this illness, and is more likely to be positive [66–70]. The PCR assay was, in fact, available in the case presented, but the availability of a PCR assay for ehrlichiosis depends on the capabilities of an individual clinical microbiology. Even if available, treatment for ehrlichiosis should be initiated before the PCR result is available. Finally, making a PCR assay for ehrlichiosis available for a more rapid diagnosis may require costly upgrading of the molecular diagnostic capabilities of the clinical microbiology laboratory.

Case with Error

This case [74] involves a 43-year-old woman who was transferred from an outside hospital to a referral medical center in early June because of possible adult respiratory distress syndrome. The patient had been in excellent health until 9 days prior to admission, when she began to have low-grade fever, chills, and headache. One week prior to admission to the referral medical center, the patient had vomited and lost consciousness. She was seen at this time at an outside hospital emergency room where she was noted to have tender postoccipital lymph nodes and a white blood count of 7,600/μL. A nurse seeing this patient at the time observed a very fine papular rash that was generalized except for the palms. Her husband remembered that he had removed a tick from her neck about 9 days earlier. The clinicians seeing this patient thought that her headache was related to her tender postoccipital lymph nodes. Therefore, the patient was sent home on oral amoxicillin for a presumed infected tick bite. The patient returned to the outside hospital because of a persistent headache as well as severe dyspnea and was admitted; this admission occurred 5 days prior to the transfer to the referral medical center. At the time of admission to the outside hospital, the patient had a fever of 40.3°C. Crackles were heard on auscultation. No rash or lymphadenopathy was noted at this time. Laboratory values included a white blood count of 6,200/μL with a left shift and a platelet count of 72,000/μL. A radiograph of the chest revealed a diffuse bilateral air-space opacification with air bronchograms, and arterial blood gases showed hypoxemia. The patient was intubated and placed on ventilatory assistance; a bronchoscopic examination was done and was normal. Cultures of the washings were negative as were blood cultures. The patient remained febrile and after 6 days of hospitalization was transferred to the referral medical center on a respirator. One dose of doxycycline was administered on the day of transfer. Despite continuation of doxycycline as well as other therapy, the patient rapidly developed cerebral edema and died within 2 days after the transfer. A serologic test on blood obtained before death, performed at the Centers for Disease Control and Prevention (CDC), revealed an elevated IgM titer of 1:2048 for *Rickettsia rickettsii*. The CDC also performed immunohistochemical staining for *R. rickettsii* on paraffin-embedded sections of brain obtained at autopsy; there was high reactivity in and around endothelial cells in the brain. A postmortem diagnosis of Rocky Mountain spotted fever (RMSF) with meningoencephalitis caused by *R. rickettsii* was made.

Explanation and Consequences

Failure to consider an uncommon infection in this case resulted in an unfortunate outcome. This case of RMSF is similar to the previously described case involving ehrlichiosis/anaplasmosis in a number of ways. In both cases, the initial failure to consider a tickborne illness in summer months [69,72,73] resulted in a delay in the diagnosis and treatment of an infection. In both cases, a tickborne illness was eventually considered; unfortunately in this case, a rickettsial meningoencephalitis resulted in death. RMSF is still the most lethal tickborne illness in the United States [74–76]. Howard T. Ricketts first described this spotted fever illness approximately 100 years ago; this illness was transmitted by Montana ticks and killed up to 75% of the patients infected [76]. Today, RMSF is more likely to be found in the southeastern United States than in the Rocky Mountains. There are a number of pitfalls related to the evaluation of the patient with possible RMSF. These include (1) waiting for the rash to develop; (2) misdiagnosing the febrile illness as another infection such as gastroenteritis; (3) discounting the diagnosis in the absence of history of tick bite; (4) using an inappropriate geographic exclusion; (5) using an inappropriate seasonal exclusion; (6) failing to treat on clinical suspicion; (7) failing to elicit an appropriate history; and (8) failing to treat with doxycycline [75]. The first opportunity for the diagnostic consideration of RMSF with initiation of empirical doxycycline therapy was at the point when the patient initially visited an emergency room. At this time, she was complaining of fever and headache and was noted to have a rash; the husband also recalled having removed a tick from her neck. This is sufficient clinical information to suspect RMSF and initiate empirical therapy with doxycycline. The diagnosis of RMSF has been, and continues to be, problematic [75,76]. The most widely used diagnostic tool is serologic testing, which is not useful during active infection. As noted with ehrlichiosis, seroconversion of RMSF infection may not occur until 3 weeks into the illness. PCR assays for diagnosing RMSF have been developed [77]; to date, these assays have not been fully evaluated in the clinical setting. A critical issue in their usefulness would be the length of time that *R. rickettsii* would remain in the blood. Of interest is a recent report of a combined PCR and electrospray ionization mass spectrometry method that was able to detect both *Ehrlichia* species and *R. rickettsii* [78]. The diagnosis and empirical doxycycline therapy of RMSF is particularly difficult in children as pediatricians, family physicians, and/or emergency room physicians may not appreciate that RMSF is seen in children [79] or be aware that the appropriate treatment strategy requires doxycycline treatment before the rash is seen [80]. For example, one study [80] found that only 21% of family practice clinicians and 25% of emergency room physicians correctly identified doxycycline as the antibiotic of choice for treating children with RMSF. Finally, it should be noted that a newly recognized tickborne spotted fever group rickettsiosis has been described [81]. The cause of this tickborne escar-associated spotted fever group rickettsiosis is *R. parkeri,* which originally was thought to be nonpathogenic in humans. Clinically, this rickettsiosis presents in a manner that is very similar to RMSF with symptoms of fever, fatigue, myalgia, headache, and a generalized rash; in addition, patients describe a "sore" or "pimple" at the site of a tick bite. This escar typically precedes the onset of fever by several days. This illness, like RMSF, is mostly seen in the southeastern Unites States. As with RMSF, empirical therapy with doxycycline should be initiated in patients with this constellation of symptoms.

Case with Error

This case [82] involves a 29-year-old man who was admitted to a medical center in the Midwest because of a 4-day history of fever, chills, headache, and neck stiffness. This was the third episode of a similar nature in the past 4 months. The patient had been treated with amoxicillin-clavulanate for the first two episodes. Additional symptoms during these previous two episodes had included arthralgias, diarrhea, and cough. Between these acute episodes of fever, chills, and headache, the patient noted fatigue, night sweats, and loss of appetite. There was no history of any insect bites. The patient's past medical history included a splenectomy 15 years earlier for a posttraumatic rupture of the spleen. A hemoglobin concentration obtained during the earlier episodes was

9.2 g/dL with a slightly elevated total bilirubin as well as slightly elevated liver enzyme levels. The physical examination of the patient revealed no hepatomegaly. At the time of admission, microscopic examination of a Giemsa-stained blood smear revealed a low number of intraerythrocytic trophozoites of *Babesia*. A classic "Maltese cross" (tetrads) was also identified. Therapy with clindamycin and quinine was initiated; the patient improved and was discharged from the hospital.

Explanation and Consequences

This case illustrates once more the failure to consider an uncommon infection leading to a medical error. Babesiosis [83,84] is another tickborne infection seen during summer months that can be particularly difficult to identify unless it is considered in the differential diagnosis [85]. Clinically, babesiosis resembles malaria and is endogenous to the United States. Observing intraerythrocytic ring-forms in a blood smear can quickly make the diagnosis if the clinician requests such smears. In this case, multiple episodes of a febrile illness went undiagnosed until a routine blood smear and an alert medical technologist allowed the diagnosis of babesiosis to be made. Other similar cases with a delayed diagnosis of babesiosis have been reported [86]. This case, like those of ehrlichiosis and RMSF, emphasizes the need to consider tickborne infections in summer months in anyone who presents with prolonged and undulating fevers, chills, headache, myalgias, and arthralgias. Moreover, this case emphasizes the need to consider intraerythrocytic parasitic infections such as babesiosis [83,84] and malaria [87,88] in patients with recurrent fevers; such patients may require the review of multiple thin and thick blood smears to make a diagnosis. The diagnosis in the previous case was a serendipitous finding on a routine blood smear. However, autoanalyzers [89] or a less observant medical technologist [90] might miss this diagnosis; multiple blood smears and/or thick smears may be required. Actually, a careful review by a medical technologist or pathologist of abnormal red blood cell images stored in current blood autoanalyzers is the best way to make a diagnosis of babesiosis, as there are far more red blood cells screened and abnormal red blood cells stored as an image than is possible with a blood smear. Finally, PCR methods have been described [91], but are not widely available. Moreover, the diagnosis must be considered before a PCR assay can be ordered.

Case with Error

This case [92] is involves a 59-year-old man who was referred to a northeastern U.S. medical center hospital in late summer because of neck pain, weakness in the right arm, and cranial-nerve palsies. The patient had been in his usual state of health until 5 weeks prior to admission when he experienced a febrile illness accompanied by neck stiffness. The patient worked as a land surveyor, lived in a wooded area, played golf, and owned dogs; he had noted tick bites in the past, but none recently. He had not noted any rashes following these tick bites. His primary care physician saw him at this time and noted thrombocytopenia on a complete blood count. The patient was treated with antibiotics with resolution of the thrombocytopenia within 2 weeks. However, the neck pain worsened and numbness and weakness of the right hand developed. An orthopedic surgeon evaluated him 4 days prior to admission; a magnetic resonance imaging (MRI) of the neck 2 days prior to admission revealed degenerative changes of the spine at multiple levels from C3 to T2 and a central herniation at the C3-C4 level. On the day before admission, the patient developed ptosis and diplopia. On the day of admission, the patient was evaluated at another hospital. He did not have fever at this time. A computed tomography scan of the head showed no abnormalities. The patient was transferred to the referral hospital at this time for a more extensive neurologic evaluation. On admission, the patient's physical examination was unremarkable except for the neurologic examination, which revealed left ptosis, asymmetric smile, weakness of both arms with 3/5 in the right wrist, absent right biceps and triceps reflexes, and a left Babinski reflex. MRI scanning of the brain showed enhancement of the bilateral fifth and bilateral third cranial nerves and evidence of microangiopathic disease. A lumbar puncture was done and revealed an elevated cell count (453 WBCs/μL with 77% lymphocytes and 19% monocytes), an elevated protein, and a normal glucose. The patient's muscle strength decreased over the first day of hospitalization; on the second day MRI scanning of the spine after administration of gadolinium revealed leptomeningeal enhancement that extended from the lower thoracic portion of the spinal cord to the roots of the cauda equina. On the third day of hospitalization, a repeat lumbar puncture revealed an elevated lymphocyte count with atypical cells of an uncertain origin; flow-cytometric analysis revealed large CD19+ and CD20- cells that lacked demonstrable surface light-chain expression, CD4+ and CD8+ cells, and polyclonal CD20+ B cells with cytoplasmic kappa and lambda light-chain expression. The patient continued to do poorly with dyspnea and dysarthria on the fourth day followed by respiratory failure on the sixth day of hospitalization. Empirical therapy with intravenous ceftriaxone was initiated on the fifth hospital day; doxycycline and acyclovir were added on the sixth day. A third lumbar puncture was done on the seventh day of hospitalization; this revealed atypical lymphocytes that were suspicious for a lymphoproliferative disorder. A PCR assay on the first sample of cerebrospinal fluid from the first day of hospitalization revealed a single, discrete rearrangement of the immunoglobulin heavy-chain gene, suspicious for the presence of a clonal B-cell population. A lymphoma was considered. The patient continued to be afebrile over the next 3 days; the neurologic deficits continued unchanged. On the 11th hospital day, the results of cerebrospinal fluid tests for *Borrelia burgdorferi* were reported as positive; these included a PCR assay as well as IgM, IgG, and IgA antibody production in the cerebrospinal fluid. In addition, a positive IgM antibody and an indeterminate IgG antibody were seen in serum and confirmed by Western blotting per the CDC-recommended 2-tiered antibody testing approach using ELISA testing followed by Western blotting [93]. This patient responded to 4 weeks of intravenous ceftriaxone and was discharged to a rehabilitation hospital for an addition 3 weeks; he is now living independently at home.

Explanation and Consequences

Failure to consider another uncommon tickborne infection led to diagnostic confusion at a number of different points in this complicated case. The first point occurred when the patient was first seen in early summer. This patient's primary care physician should have considered tickborne infections in the differential diagnosis for a febrile illness in a patient with thrombocytopenia. The second point occurred after the patient experienced continued neck pain despite the response to antimicrobial therapy. This was followed by numbness and weakness of the right arm; this plus the ptosis and diplopia should have prompted serologic testing for Lyme disease [94,95]. As the laboratory diagnosis of early Lyme disease has been and continues to be problematic [96–98], empirical continuation of the initial antimicrobial therapy [99] could have been done while serologic testing for Lyme was being done (and repeated if negative). As the diagnosis of Lyme disease is generally based on serologic testing, a delay in the patient's antibody response to the infection can result in a delay in the diagnosis. Early Lyme disease is particularly difficult to diagnose and empirical antimicrobial therapy should be considered with the appropriate clinical situation [99]. The patient in this case was eventually hospitalized for a neurologic evaluation that included a lumbar puncture. At this point, the diagnostic confusion in this case was due to the presence of large B cells in the cerebrospinal fluid, which raised the possibility of a B-cell lymphoma [100]. However, antigenic stimulus due to *B. burgdorferi* infection is known to cause a blastoid transformation of B and T lymphocytes that can result in cerebrospinal fluid cytology mimicking central nervous system malignancy [101,102]. In this case, broad-spectrum empirical antimicrobial therapy, which included intravenous ceftriaxone, eventually resulted in resolution of this patient's neuroborreliosis.

Case with Error

This case [103] involves a 65-year-old man of Indian origin who was transferred to a neurologic unit in a medical center for the evaluation of neck stiffness, fever, and drowsiness. This patient had been admitted to the referring hospital 10 days previously because of a 4-week history of abdominal pain and diarrhea. An extensive evaluation including sigmoidoscopy and evaluation of stool samples for ova and parasites had not revealed a cause for the abdominal pain and diarrhea. This patient's past medical history was significant for giant cell arteritis diagnosed 2 months previously; the patient had responded nicely to prednisolone therapy. The patient had lived in England for many years, but had returned to India for a brief visit several years previously. On admission, the patient was unconscious, but responded to painful stimuli. His vital signs included a temperature of 38.5°C, pulse of 100 bpm, and respiratory rate at 32/minute. The patient was noted to have marked neck stiffness and a positive Kernig's sign. The patient's abdomen was diffusely tender; the remainder of the physical examination was unremarkable. Laboratory values included a white blood cell count of 8,900/µL with 90% neutrophils, 7% lymphocytes, 2% monocytes, and 1% eosinophils. A chest radiograph that had been normal 1 week previously revealed patchy infiltrates in both lung fields. A lumbar puncture demonstrated cloudy cerebrospinal fluid with a Gram stain revealing many gram-negative bacilli. The cerebrospinal fluid white blood cell count was 900/µL with 80% neutrophils; the protein concentration was elevated while the glucose concentration was low. The patient was quickly treated with antimicrobial agents for presumed bacterial meningitis based upon this clinical presentation; the diagnosis was confirmed by positive cerebrospinal fluid cultures for *Escherichia coli*. Blood and urine cultures revealed no growth. The patient did not respond to this antimicrobial therapy; 24 hours later a sputum examination revealed *Strongyloides stercoralis* larvae. A diagnosis of systemic strongyloidosis was made, and intravenous thiabendazole was started. *S. stercoralis* larvae were subsequently noted in the stool and urine. Despite the addition of thiabendazole to this patient's therapy, the patient continued to deteriorate further over the following week and finally died.

Explanation and Consequences

Failure to consider an uncommon parasitic infection such as disseminated strongyloidosis that may present with concomitant gram-negative meningitis might seem to be a rare event. However, the failure to consider such disseminated strongyloidosis infections is not an isolated occurrence and has been reported for *E. coli* meningitis [103,104] as well as gram-negative sepsis with acute respiratory failure [105,106]. The capacity of strongyloides to replicate, hyperinfect, and disseminate in the human host is limited and rarely happens. The use of corticosteroids, as reported in this case [103], is the most commonly reported risk factor for disseminated strongyloidosis [107,108]. Steroid-induced immunosuppression has been reported to cause activation of strongyloides, resulting in increased egg production. It also has been suggested that corticosteroids may increase ecdysteroid-like substances in the intestinal wall; these naturally occurring sterols then act as molting signals leading to increased numbers of autoinfective filariform larvae [109]. In addition, corticosteroids are known to reduce the eosinophil count and to inhibit the mast cell response [110]. Complete blood counts during hyperinfection often show a suppression of eosinophilic count, which eliminates a potential clue. Patients who present with a peripheral eosinophilia appear to have a better prognosis, which may be related to more rapid diagnosis. Disseminated strongyloidosis is often complicated by infections caused by gut flora that cross the intestinal barrier with the invading filariform larvae. Up to 45% of systemic strongyloidosis cases are complicated by gram-negative septicemia and systemic bacterial infections have been reported in approximately 60% of cases. Clearly the manifestations and diagnosis of strongyloidosis must be considered in patients from endemic areas who are taking corticosteroids or are in other ways immunosuppressed. Strongyloidosis is a diagnostically elusive disease even in the 21st century, with delayed diagnosis still being reported [111].

Case with Averted Error

This case [112] involves a 60-year-old woman who was referred to a tertiary medical center in the northeastern United States because of fever. She had been well until 6 years previously, when she had the onset of arthralgias in multiple joints. She had been treated for these arthralgias with aspirin and indomethacin. Six months prior to admission, she had the onset of fever and chills that occurred twice monthly and then increased in frequency. During the 2 months before admission, she had fever and chills at night as often as three times per week; she also noted fatigue and malaise during this time. Her past medical history was remarkable for her husband being treated for pulmonary tuberculosis 34 years earlier. The patient denied any rash, chest pain, cough, anorexia, abdominal pain, or weight loss. On physical examination, a firm, mobile lymph node was felt in the right axilla. The tip of the spleen was felt, and the liver edge was palpated 2 cm below the right costal margin. The remainder of the physical examination was unremarkable. Initial laboratory values were normal. The patient was afebrile on admission, but on the fourth hospital day became febrile to 39°C; then 2 days later the temperature rose to 39.4°C and was accompanied by a shaking chill. A biopsy of the right axillary lymph node was performed and revealed noncaseating granulomatous lymphadenitis with Schaumann bodies. Acid-fast and silver-methenamine stains for mycobacteria and fungi were negative; cultures of the lymph node also yielded no growth. The lymph node biopsy suggested a diagnosis of sarcoidosis although the patient had no pulmonary findings consistent with this disease. She was discharged at this time only to be readmitted 3.5 months later with continued fever, chills, and night sweats. She also noted weight loss over this time period. Physical examination at this time revealed lymphadenopathy in both axillae as well as in the right supraclavicular area, but was otherwise unremarkable. The temperature ranged as high as 38.3°C daily. Laboratory values and chest and abdominal x-rays were unchanged from the first admission. The working diagnosis at this time was fever of unknown origin. An upper gastrointestinal series and small bowel study were negative as was a barium-enema examination. Mild hepatosplenomegaly was noted, and lymphoma was considered as a possible diagnosis. On the 14th hospital day, an exploratory laparotomy was done; this revealed extensive lymphadenopathy at the base of the small-bowel mesentery. A biopsy of one of the lymph nodes revealed granulomas with large macrophages with clear cytoplasm in which there was an enormous amount of periodic acid-Schiff (PAS)—positive material. These findings were consistent with Whipple's disease. A subsequently obtained peroral jejunal biopsy specimen was examined under electron microscopy and demonstrated bacillary bodies in the lamina propria outside the cells as well as intact bacillary bodies within macrophages. These electron-microscopic findings confirmed the diagnosis of Whipple's disease.

Explanation and Consequences

The delay in the diagnosis of this case of Whipple's disease was, in part, due to its somewhat atypical presentation of fever and arthralgias in a woman and, in part, due to its being a rare systemic disorder. Whipple's disease is caused by *Tropheryma whippelii*, which is an actinomycete that is difficult to culture [113]; cultures are not readily available in most clinical microbiology laboratories. These rare chronic infections classically involve the gastrointestinal tract [114], and patients typically present with diarrhea and malabsorption [115–117]. Moreover, Whipple's disease is predominantly seen in middle-aged white males, with only 12% of reported cases being seen in women. A variety of other clinical manifestations can be seen and include involvement of heart, lungs, or central nervous system. In particular, Whipple's disease can mimic sarcoidosis [118,119], as it did in this case. Indeed, the diagnosis of Whipple's disease has always been difficult [112, 115–119]. The cultivation of *T. whippelii* [113] has greatly increased the knowledge of this disorder as well as the allowing of diagnostic PCR testing [120–122]. For example, the classic form of Whipple's disease, which is characterized by PAS-positive-stained bacilli in infected small-bowel macrophages [114], represents only one form of this rare disease. This bacterium also is capable of causing localized infections such as endocarditis and meningoencephalitis [117]. Additionally, 1% to 26% of all individuals are asymptomatic carriers of this microorganism [121, 123]. Diagnostic tests for Whipple's disease currently include histopathologic staining with PAS [114,115], PCR and quantitative PCR testing [120,122], and Western blot; the diagnostic strategy can be complex and often requires interpretation [122].

STANDARDS OF CARE

▩ Failure to consider uncommon infections clearly can result in harm to a patient; it may be less clear that a medical error has occurred although the patient and/or a lawyer would likely consider such a failure to be a medical error.

▩ Failure to consider uncommon infections as a source of medical errors can be avoided by a number of mechanisms; these include use of the medical literature [124], use of the Internet (eg, PubMed [125] or *UpToDate* [126]), consultation with the clinical microbiology laboratory director [127], and consultation with an infectious diseases clinician [128,129].

▩ Tickborne infections are an emerging infectious threat [73] and cause uncommon infections that must be considered in the differential diagnosis of febrile patients seen during summer months in order to avoid medical errors.

▩ Broad-spectrum empirical antimicrobial therapy may be needed while the differential diagnosis is being developed and the results of diagnostic testing are pending; this is particularly true for tickborne infections where only babesiosis can be quickly diagnosed.

▩ Uncommon infections that are difficult to diagnose such as parasitic diseases and Whipple's disease are often diagnostic problems that require infectious diseases consultation [108,122,128,129].

FAILURE TO APPRECIATE THE PROPER TIMING FOR SEROLOGY TESTS

> Failure to appreciate the proper timing for serology is another common medical error and leads to confusion when the "obvious" diagnosis is "ruled out" by the serologic test. Consultation with the laboratory can assist with this problem.

Case with Error

This case [130] involves a 70-year-old African American woman with end-stage renal disease secondary to hypertension who had received a deceased-donor kidney transplant 6 years prior to being transferred from another hospital for the present tertiary care center admission. Her graft function had been stable with a serum creatinine of 2 mg/dL; her maintenance immunosuppressive therapy consisted of 5 mg prednisone per day, 750 mg mycophenolate mofetil twice a day, and 50 mg cyclosporine A twice a day. She had been in her usual state of health until 3 days prior to the transfer when she presented to another hospital with new onset fever as well as nausea, vomiting, and abdominal pain of 2 weeks' duration. A white blood cell count was slightly elevated. She was initially treated with broad-spectrum antimicrobial therapy; she developed confusion and tonic-clonic seizures over the next 2 days despite the antimicrobial therapy. A computed tomography scan of the head was normal. A lumbar puncture revealed a leukocyte count of 21 cells/μL with 83% lymphocytes and normal protein and glucose levels. Parenteral acyclovir was started, and she was transferred to the tertiary care medical center. Upon arrival, the patient was stuporous and had a temperature of 102.8°F. Myoclonic movements of the upper extremities were noted on physical examination. The patient was treated with only intravenous acyclovir for possible herpes simplex meningoencephalitis. A repeat computed tomography scan and a magnetic resonance imaging scan of the head were done and reported as normal. A second lumbar puncture done 3 days after the first revealed a continued lymphocytosis (99%) and an increase in the protein level to 130 mg/dL. Acyclovir was continued, and broad-spectrum antimicrobial agents were added. Bacterial and viral cultures of the cerebrospinal fluid were negative as were blood cultures. PCR for HSV, VZV, and CMV in the cerebrospinal fluid were negative. CSF serology was done for California encephalitis , eastern equine encephalitis, St. Louis encephalitis, and West Nile encephalitis; all were negative. The patient's fever resolved after 14 days, and all antimicrobial agents were discontinued. The etiology of this acute encephalitis was undiagnosed. The patient continued to have seizure activity and required tracheostomy for respiratory support. She was transferred to a subacute care facility where convalescent serology was done. The results for West Nile virus are summarized. On days 2 and 5, West Nile virus-specific IgM by capture EIA from cerebrospinal fluid were done and were negative. However, convalescent serum samples from days 25 and 42 were positive for West Nile virus IgM and IgG. A diagnosis of West Nile virus encephalitis was made.

Explanation and Consequences

This case illustrates the need for proper timing of serologic testing. Acute West Nile encephalitis is a serious public health issue in the United States with over 700 cases reported to the Centers for Disease Control and Prevention (CDC) in 2009 [131]. The CDC recommends that West Nile virus IgM detection by an IgM capture ELISA assay in serum or cerebrospinal fluid should be the major laboratory tool used to identify symptomatic patients with acute West Nile virus infections. This test has a sensitivity approaching 100% in appropriately timed samples. In early symptomatic infections, the West Nile virus can be detected by PCR in serum or cerebrospinal fluid [132]. However, levels of West Nile virus RNA typically peak before symptoms appear and then rapidly decline as IgM antibody production begins [133]. Thus, there is a limited window for RNA detection. Once IgM antibodies for West Nile virus appear, they remain detectable for several months after the acute illness [134]. Although most patients with West Nile virus encephalitis present late in their illness, some patients seeking medical assistance within a week of symptom onset may still be in the RNA-positive/antibody-negative window and be missed if only IgM testing is done. To avoid missing cases of acute West Nile infection, both West Nile virus RNA testing and West Nile virus IgM testing may be required [135]. As there is no current antiviral therapy for West Nile virus encephalitis [136], a delay in the diagnosis as seen in this case is not a therapeutic problem.

Case with Averted Error

This case [137] involves a 10-year-old boy who was admitted to a children's hospital after 2 days of fever (38.5°C), disorientation, vomiting, and diarrhea. Examination of motor, sensory, cerebellar function, and gait on admission were all normal. A lumbar puncture obtained on admission revealed 135 leukocytes/μL with 97% lymphocytes. The cerebrospinal protein level was elevated, and the glucose level was normal. Cerebrospinal fluid Gram stain, bacterial and viral cultures, and herpes simplex PCR were all negative. A brain magnetic resonance imaging (MRI) study done on admission and repeated on day 3 were both normal. The electroencephalogram (EEG) done on day 2 demonstrated intermittent focal slowing over the left temporo-occipital region. The child received a 10-day intravenous course of acyclovir and improved over this time. He was discharged following this course of acyclovir. Two days later, he had seizure activity and was readmitted. On physical examination, the child was postictal and aphasic. Seizures were controlled with phenytoin. A head computed tomography scan with contrast revealed generalized enhancement of the meninges. A lumbar puncture revealed 128 leukocytes/μL with 89% lymphocytes; the protein and glucose levels were elevated. All cerebrospinal fluid cultures were again negative; PCR for herpes simplex was also negative. A brain MRI at this time demonstrated abnormal signal intensity bilaterally in cortical and subcortical regions in the frontal-temporal lobe. The EEG showed periodic lateralizing epileptic discharges over the left frontocentral-temporal region. Parenteral acyclovir was reinitiated and continued for an additional 14 days. Serologic studies were negative for eastern equine encephalitis, western equine encephalitis, St. Louis encephalitis, California encephalitis, and herpes simplex virus. However, serologic testing for La Crosse virus is summarized. The serum hemagglutination titer for

La Crosse virus was 1:10 on the day of admission and 1:160 on day 16 after readmission. A diagnosis of La Crosse viral encephalitis was made. The child was discharged and has been well with no long-term sequelae from this encephalitis.

Explanation and Consequences

This case illustrates the delayed diagnosis of viral encephalitis due to the normal delay in the host antibody response to infection by the La Crosse virus. La Crosse virus is a mosquito-borne arbovirus that is the primary cause of pediatric encephalitis in the United States [138]. Usually this encephalitis is mild with minimal neurologic sequelae although more severe infections have been reported [137,139]. La Crosse virus encephalitis can be difficult to distinguish clinically from other viral infections of the CNS, and specific laboratory testing is required. In general, a viral-specific IgM antibody capture enzyme immunoassay done on cerebrospinal fluid is the preferred diagnostic test for La Crosse encephalitis [140]. Serum IgM antibody levels of La Crosse virus may remain elevated for almost 1 year in over half of patients; serologic diagnosis, therefore, requires demonstration of a fourfold or greater change in serum antibody titer [141]. This criterion was met in this case. As no treatment is available for this infection, delay in diagnosis is not clinically important. The authors, however, point out that prolonged therapy with acyclovir for a presumed diagnosis of herpes simplex viral encephalitis could have been avoided if a PCR test for La Crosse virus were readily available. Such PCR tests have been developed [142], but have not been clinically validated and thus are not readily available in most clinical microbiology laboratories.

Case with Averted Error

This case [143] involves a 2-year-old girl who presented to a tertiary referral center in the Northeast with a 6-week history of multiple, persistent, erythematous, ringlike lesions and recurrent fever. There was no history of a tick bite. Three weeks into the illness, the child's pediatrician had seen her and ordered a serologic test for *Borrelia burgdorferi* (ELISA IgM and IgG); this serology was negative. At this point of the illness, the pediatrician considered Lyme disease to be excluded because of the negative serology for *B. burgdorferi*, and the child was not treated. However, the child returned because of these persistent skin lesions, which were consistent with multiple erythema migrans. Therefore, the serologic test for Lyme disease was repeated. At this time, which was 6 weeks into the illness, the serology was ELISA IgG positive for *B. burgdorferi* at a titer of 1:2560 and ELISA IgM negative. A Western blot for *B. burgdorferi* was also positive and thus confirmed this diagnosis. The child was successfully treated with amoxicillin.

Explanation and Consequences

This case nicely illustrates the failure to appreciate the proper timing for the serologic diagnosis of Lyme disease. The child's pediatrician recognized that this child had erythematous skin lesions that might represent erythema migrans [144,145] and thus considered Lyme disease as a diagnosis. Moreover, multifocal lesions as seen in this case are recognized as representing an early stage of systemic infection [146]. The initial error made by the pediatrician was in failing to appreciate that serology might not allow the diagnosis of early Lyme disease [97–99]. Fortunately, the child returned because of the persistent multiple erythema migrans and was successfully treated. Suspicion of Lyme disease based on erythema migrans is sufficient reason to begin empiric antimicrobial therapy [99,144].

Case with Averted Error

This case [147] involves a 41-year-old man who was hospitalized for the evaluation of acute jaundice. This patient had no significant past medical history and had been well until 5 days before admission, when he suddenly had fever, chill, nausea, and vomiting. Two days before admission, he noticed that his urine had become darker in color and that his stools were lighter in color. On the day of admission, he noticed that his sclerae were yellow. He contacted his family physician and subsequently was admitted to the hospital for the evaluation of acute jaundice. His only risk factor for jaundice elicited in his history of present illness was that he owned six hound dogs that frequently urinated inside his home. The patient admitted that he would often clean up this urine and then fail to wash his hands before eating. On physical examination, the patient was jaundiced and had a fever of 101.1°F. His sclerae were icteric, but without conjunctival injection. Laboratory values included an elevated white blood cell count of 15,800/μL with a left shift and an elevated serum creatinine of 4.6 mg/dL. Liver function studies revealed the following values: total bilirubin 24.9 mg/dL, direct bilirubin 21.6 mg/dL, alkaline phosphatase 132U/L, AST 125U/L, and ALT 76U/L. Results of serologic tests for hepatitis A and B were negative; a biliary sonogram was normal. An infectious diseases consultation was obtained; a presumptive diagnosis of icteric leptospirosis (Weil's syndrome) was made based upon the clinical picture and the exposure to canine urine [148]. Empiric antimicrobial therapy with intravenous penicillin G was initiated. The patient did not require dialysis; after several days, the serum creatinine began to decline. On the eighth day of illness, conjunctival suffusion developed. On the 10th day, the intravenous penicillin was stopped and oral tetracycline was started. Blood and urine cultures revealed no growth. On the 12th day, the patient complained of a severe headache and became acutely disoriented. A lumbar puncture was done and revealed unremarkable cerebrospinal fluid. This episode was thought to represent aseptic meningitis, which is a known complication during the second (immunogenic) stage of leptospirosis [149]. The patient recovered from this episode and was discharged. Serologic testing for the microscopic agglutination titers for leptospirosis is summarized. The patient's serum microscopic agglutination titers on admission were 1:12 and on day 18 were 1:500.

Explanation and Consequences

Leptospirosis is a zoonotic disease caused by the spirochetes of the genus *Leptospira* and is considered to be one of the most common zoonoses in the world [147–150]. In the past decade, leptospirosis has been recognized as an emerging public health problem that occurs in urban and rural areas of developing and developed countries [150,151]. Humans are accidental hosts and become infected through exposure to environmental sources contaminated by the urine of chronically infected mammals. In the United States, the most common sources of exposure are dogs, livestock, and wild animals, especially rodents. Outbreaks of leptospirosis have been reported and are often due to natural disasters such as floods [152]. Leptospirosis is also recognized as an infection seen in returned travelers from the tropics [153,154]. Hospitalized cases of leptospirosis may have mortality rates as high as 25%; this is, in part, related to a delay in diagnosis. The majority of leptospirosis cases are diagnosed by serology. The current standard is the microscopic agglutination test, which involves the reaction of antigens in the form of live *Leptospira* organisms with the antibodies found in the patient's sera. A positive reaction results in agglutination of the *Leptospira* that can be seen microscopically. The IgG antibody response to leptospirosis to this test takes about 2 weeks and can be delayed by antimicrobial therapy. In this case, the clinical suspicion was high, and empiric antimicrobial therapy was started. The serologic diagnosis was made on day 18, which is typical for the diagnosis of leptospirosis. There are new serologic methods that are commercially available [155]; some of these tests measure an IgM response and may thus allow more rapid results. PCR testing is also being developed [156] and should allow the most rapid means of diagnosis.

Case with Averted Error

This case [157] involves a 2-year-old previously healthy boy who was admitted with a history of high fever and a "lump" on his right hip area for 2 days. The child had been limping and favored his right leg. Physical examination revealed an elevated temperature of 39.5°C. A tentative diagnosis of septic arthritis or acute osteomyelitis of the right hip was made. Tenderness was elicited on moving the right hip, but no "lump" was noted. Otherwise, the physical examination was unremarkable. Laboratory studies were also unremarkable and included a normal hematologic profile as well as a normal erythrocyte sedimentation rate of 22 mm/hour. A radiograph of the right hip and a gallium citrate-67 bone scan were done; both were normal. A *Brucella* agglutination titer was done and reported as negative. Blood cultures obtained on admission revealed no growth. Aspiration of the right hip on admission was cultured; the routine bacterial cultures were negative. The child was discharged with a diagnosis of transient viral synovitis. Two weeks later, the child was still febrile and limping. Although a *Brucella* culture of the right-hip aspirate had not been ordered, the microbiologist had noted the clinical data on the requisition form and thus had included a *Brucella* culture; this culture was now positive. A diagnosis of brucellosis was made, and the child was successfully treated.

Explanation and Consequences

Brucellosis is another zoonotic disease [158] for which the clinical diagnosis remains a considerable challenge to clinicians and laboratories alike [159,160]. In particular, the frequent presentation of brucellosis as a nonspecific febrile illness in adults and children (so-called periodic or undulant fever) and its ability to infect virtually any organ or tissue has resulted in this infection being described as a "disease of mistakes" [160]. Culture of *Brucella* species is the definitive diagnosis and is considered the gold standard in the laboratory diagnosis of brucellosis; unfortunately, culture is both laborious [161] and hazardous [162]. For example, optimal cultivation of *Brucella* species requires biphasic Ruiz-Castaneda bottles and 6 weeks of incubation time; the yield is 40% to 90% in acute cases and 5% to 20% in chronic cases [160,161]. Commercial automated blood culture systems are capable of isolating *Brucella* species [163], but bacteremia in brucellosis is also known to be unpredictable [164]. Therefore, serological assays are the most commonly relied upon diagnostic test for brucellosis [160,165]. In the previous case, the serologic assay was negative. Had the microbiologist not specifically done cultures for *Brucella* species, the diagnosis would have been missed during this admission and thus delayed. As this case seemed to represent an acute case of brucellosis, the serologic assay would likely have become positive in time. An 11-month delay in the diagnosis of *Brucella* septic arthritis of the knee has been reported; reconstruction with bone grafts was required in this case [166]. Although brucellosis is not a common problem in the United States, *Brucella suis* infections associated with feral swine hunting have been reported [167]. Clinicians treating patients with undiagnosed febrile illness should consider brucellosis; the limitations of serologic testing must be appreciated.

STANDARDS OF CARE

■ Certain infectious diseases such as many viral infections, as well as infections involving *Mycoplasma, Leptospira, Borrelia, Treponema, Brucella, Coxiella,* and *Chlamydia,* often require a serologic diagnosis; appreciation of the time required for an antibody response to the acute infection is important when obtaining such serologic tests.

■ Failure to appreciate the proper timing for serology tests can result in harm to a patient even though the correct diagnosis was considered, and an appropriate serology test was ordered; failure to appreciate the proper timing for serology tests is a subtle but real form of medical error.

■ Unlike failure to consider infection or failure to consider uncommon infections, in this situation the correct infection was considered; using empirical antimicrobial therapy when applicable can avoid this type of medical error.

■ Appreciating the appropriate timing of serology tests may result in repeating a serology test that is initially negative; empirical antimicrobial therapy as mentioned earlier prevents harm to the patient.

FAILURE TO APPRECIATE THE SENSITIVITY OR SPECIFICITY OF MICROBIOLOGY TESTS

▶ Failure to appreciate the sensitivity or specificity of microbiology tests is another common problem and can lead to medical errors. This problem often can be avoided by consultation with the laboratory.

Case with Error

This case [168] involves a 29-year-old man who in July 2009 was transferred to the critical care unit of a tertiary medical center in the Northeast because of fever and respiratory failure. The patient had been well until 9 days earlier, when he developed a nonproductive cough and myalgias in his legs. One week earlier, he had a fever of 39.4°C; sore throat and nasal congestion then developed. The patient noted mild chest pain during expiration; his cough became productive of clear sputum. He was seen at the emergency room of another hospital 4 days before admission and was found to be in mild distress; his temperature was 38.2°C and his pulse was 106 bpm. Influenza was considered; a raid test of a buccal swab specimen was negative for influenza A and B antigens. The patient was given intravenous ceftriaxone and discharged home on oral doxycycline. He returned to the same emergency room on the next afternoon because of persistent fever, cough, and myalgias. The temperature was 39°C; rhonchi were noted in the left lower lung field. A chest radiograph revealed incomplete segmental consolidation of the apical posterior segment of the right upper lobe suggesting pneumonia. Levofloxacin was prescribed, and he was sent home. Two days later, the patient again returned to the same emergency room. This time, he was still febrile; his respiratory rate was 34 breaths/minute and his oxygen saturation 88% while he was breathing 4 L oxygen by nasal cannula. A chest radiograph showed progression of the right upper lobe process as well as patchy air-space disease in the right lower lobe and the middle and lower lobes on the left side. He was admitted to the hospital where his respiratory distress worsened over the next

14 hours despite broad-spectrum antimicrobial therapy. He was then transferred to the critical care unit of a nearby tertiary care medical center. There he was continued on broad-spectrum antimicrobial agents and was also treated with oseltamivir for the novel 2009 H1N1 influenza virus that was known to be in circulation. PCR testing performed at the state laboratory confirmed the diagnosis of the 2009 H1N1 influenza A virus. Despite therapy with oseltamivir and supportive critical care management, the patient expired on the ninth hospital day.

Explanation and Consequences

In this case, the negative testing for influenza virus on the buccal swab done during the first visit to an emergency room did not rule out 2009 H1N1 influenza virus infection in this patient because such rapid diagnostic tests for influenza have low sensitivity [169,170]. This case occurred in the summer of 2009. During the spring of 2009, this novel influenza A (H1N1) virus of swine origin emerged in humans in North America and thus was considered a possibility during the first visit of this patient to an emergency room. Indeed, a rapid influenza test was done at this first visit. However, the sensitivity of rapid diagnostic tests for influenza during the peak influenza season is approximately 60%; a lower prevalence of influenza at other times of the year will result in a lower sensitivity for rapid influenza testing. It is thus not surprising that the rapid test was negative in this case. Moreover, buccal swabs are not ideal for influenza testing; nasopharyngeal swabs are preferred. Finally, empiric antiviral treatment should be based on the clinical picture rather than the results of rapid influenza testing. The Infectious Diseases Society of America Clinical Practice Guidelines currently recommends early treatment (ideally within 48 hours) with oseltamivir or zanamivir for persons highly suspected of influenza virus infection [171]. Such empiric antiviral treatment might have made a difference in this case, but was not recommended by the CDC in early summer of 2009 [172].

Case with Averted Error

This case [173] involves a 46-year-old male with a cystopleural shunt *in situ* for 14 months as palliative treatment of a spinal arachnoid cyst who was admitted to the hospital because of progressive worsening of lower limb weakness. This patient had initially been seen for a similar complaint of progressive weakness in the lower limbs and had been diagnosed with an intradural extramedullary cystic lesion anterior to the spinal cord for which a cystopleural shunt had been inserted. This shunt had resulted in substantial improvement, and the patient had been able to walk unaided. However, 14 months after insertion of this shunt, there was a recurrence of bilateral lower limb weakness. On admission to the hospital, the patient was afebrile and had normal vital signs. Physical examination on admission demonstrated decreased lower limb power and upper motor neuron signs. A magnetic resonance imaging study revealed nodular thickened leptomeningeal enhancement in the thoracic spine as well as a right pleural effusion. Laboratory values included a complete blood count, liver function studies, and renal function studies; all were within normal limits. The cystopleural shunt was taped; the cerebrospinal fluid was clear and colorless. The initial analysis of the cerebrospinal fluid demonstrated a total cell count of 93/μL (36% neutrophils, 30% lymphocytes, and 34% mononuclear cells), an elevated protein level, and a normal glucose level. These findings suggested chronic meningitis. However, Gram stain, Ziehl Neelsen acid-fast staining, Indian ink examination, and PCR for *Mycobacterium tuberculosis* were all negative. A cryptococcal antigen test (CALAS®, Meridian Bioscience Inc., Cincinnati, Ohio) was done on both the patient's serum and cerebrospinal fluid; both were negative. Culture of the cerebrospinal fluid was negative for bacteria and fungi. Because of the cerebrospinal fluid changes suggesting chronic meningitis, cerebrospinal fluid was inoculated into the BACTEC™ Myco/F Lytic bottle (Becton Dickinson, Sparks, Maryland). Growth was detected after 6 days of incubation; subcultures revealed a small colony variant of *Cryptococcus neoformans*. A diagnosis of cryptococcal meningitis was made. Fenestration of the spinal arachnoid cyst and removal of the shunt was performed along with a 6-week course of intravenous amphotericin B and intravenous flucytosine. This intravenous therapy was followed by oral fluconazole. Cerebrospinal fluid cultures were negative for *Cryptococcus neoformans* after 8 weeks of therapy.

Explanation and Consequences

In this case, both the cryptococcal antigen test and the cerebrospinal cultures initially were negative in this nonimmunosuppressed patient. Clearly there was an opportunity for a medical error to occur had the patient been discharged without determining the cause of his chronic meningitis. The cerebrospinal fluid findings of chronic meningitis prompted additional cultures using a more sensitive culture method (BACTEC™ Myco/F Lytic bottle) because both clinicians and microbiologists recognized the limitations of the cryptococcal antigen testing as well as the limitations of crytococcal cerebrospinal fluid cultures [174–176]. In particular, capsule-deficient isolates of *Cryptococcus neoformans* as seen in this case are known to cause difficulty in diagnosing chronic cryptococcal meningitis using the cerebrospinal fluid cryptococcal latex agglutination test [177]. In nonimmunosuppressed patients, the delayed diagnosis of cryptococcal meningitis is a recognized problem that has increased the morbidity and mortality of this condition [178]. Finally, false-positive cryptococcal antigen testing has been reported [179] and must be considered in such antigen testing.

Case with Error

This case [180] involves a 67-year-old woman who was admitted to the hospital for suspected pneumonia. This patient suffered from biopsy-proven sarcoidosis as well as systemic lupis erythematosus with progressive renal failure. A computer tomography scan of the chest had been done because of a weight loss of 30 lb within the last 6 months; this revealed small cystic lesions in the left lower lobe. On admission, a chest radiograph also demonstrated bilateral infiltrates of the lung as well as pleural effusions. She was admitted to the hospital and treated with ceftriaxone and clarithromycin for suspected pneumonia and initially improved on this therapy. However, microbiological evaluation including sputum culture, blood cultures, and pleural fluid cultures were negative as was a urinary antigen test for *Legionella pneumophila* (NOW® *Legionella* Urinary Antigen Test, Binax, Inc, Scarborough, Maine). The clarithromycin therapy was discontinued based upon the negative result for the urinary antigen test for *L. pneumophila* although the ceftriaxone therapy was continued. Two days later, the pulmonary function worsened and corticosteroids were added for suspected reactivation of sarcoidosis. Ceftriaxone was replaced after 12 days by piperacillin/tazobactram for suspected superinfection. Despite this broad-spectrum antimicrobial therapy along with corticosteroid therapy, the patient's clinical signs and symptoms deteriorated with the C-reactive protein and white blood count rising; the patient required emergency intubation because of acute respiratory distress syndrome. A computed tomography scan of the chest demonstrated progressing infiltrates of both lungs. The piperacillin/tazobactram was switched to meropenem; a lung biopsy was done and revealed interstitial fibrosing pneumonia with accumulation of intra-alveolar foamy macrophages. A few colonies of *Aspergillus fumigatus* initially grew from this biopsy; amphotericin B was added to the antimicrobial therapy. Despite this therapy, respiratory failure developed. A repeat chest radiograph and computed tomography of the chest demonstrated new cavitary lesions in the right upper lobe. A serologic test for *L. pneumophila* (*Legionella pneumophila* IFA, Meridian Bioscience, Cincinnati, Ohio) was done and the urinary antigen for *L. pneumophila* was repeated; both were negative. However, *L. bozemanii* grew from cultures of the lung biopsy and the Dieterle stain demonstrated intra- and extracellular rods. Clarithromycin therapy was restarted, but the patient died 2 days later.

Explanation and Consequences

Legionella species are important causes of pneumonia in humans; however, the diagnosis of *Legionella* infection is limited by the non-specific nature of clinical features and the shortcomings of diagnostic tests [181]. Currently there are more than 50 species of *Legionella* with at least 24 of these associated with human disease. Although *L. pneumophila* appears to be more pathogenic to humans and causes the majority of human disease [182], other species clearly can infect humans [183]. Importantly, cavitary pulmonary infection as seen in this case has been associated with *L. bozemanii* [184]. *L. micdadei* and *L. longbeachae* are other common etiologic agents causing human infection. Unfortunately, no single microbiology test is able to diagnose *Legionella* infection in a timely fashion with a high degree of sensitivity and specificity [181]. Although *Legionella* culture remains the most useful single test, culture diagnosis requires special media, adequate processing of specimens, and technical expertise. The standard medium used to culture *Legionella* species is buffered charcoal yeast extract (BYCE) agar. Supplementation of BYCE agar with bovine serum albumin will enhance the growth of some *Legionella* species such as *L. bozemanii* and *L. micdadei*; in contrast, addition of cefamandole to this agar as is often done will inhibit growth of these two species. Despite the appropriate use of BYCE agar for sputum cultures, the sensitivity of expectorated sputum cultures ranges from 10% to 80% as fewer than one-half of patients with *Legionella* pneumonia produce sputum. Bronchoscopy or pulmonary biopsy specimens (as in this case) are more likely to yield positive cultures than are expectorated sputum samples. The detection of soluble *Legionella* antigen in urine specimens has become a rapid and reliable tool for the diagnosis of *L. pneumophila* infections [185]. These urinary antigen tests have sensitivities in the range of 70% to 100%, but are only able to detect *L. pneumophila* serogroup 1. As seen in this case, other species of *Legionella* are not reliably detected. False-positive results for the *Legionella* urinary antigen have been reported as well [186]. Serologic testing for *Legionella* infection is hampered by the delay in seroconversion, which may take several weeks, as well as by the inability of serologic testing to accurately detect all *Legionella* species and subgroups [181]. Clearly, there remains a role for *Legionella* cultures obtained by bronchoscopy or pulmonary biopsy.

Case with Averted Error

This case [187] involves a 55-year-old immunocompromised woman who was admitted to the hospital for the evaluation of pneumonia. This patient was being treated with immunosuppressive drugs for hypoplastic myelodysplastic syndrome. Her initial pulmonary evaluation included a fine-needle lung biopsy with cultures done under computed tomography guidance as well as blood cultures; these were negative. Twice-weekly screening for circulating *Aspergillus* galactomannan (Platelia *Aspergillus* Test, Bio-Rad, Marnes-La-Coquette, France) was ordered; the result of the first screening test was negative. Empirical therapy with ceftazidime and amikacin was initiated and later switched to imipenem. However, this patient then developed a painful skin nodule of the left leg; a biopsy of this nodule revealed only necrotic tissue. Because of this skin nodule, her antimicrobial therapy was again switched to intravenous amoxicillin-clavulanic acid. Shortly after the initiation of the amoxicillin-clavulanic acid, the circulating *Aspergillus* galactomannan test became positive and remained so until 10 days following discontinuation of the amoxicillin-clavulanic acid. Although the patient had clinical findings (lung infiltrate and skin lesion) consistent with invasive *Aspergillus* infection, antifungal therapy was not done due to a previous report of false-positive galactomannan tests with piperacillin-tazobactam [188]. Instead, this group directly tested amoxicillin-clavulanic acid using vials taken directly from the hospital pharmacy. These were also positive for galactomannan. The patient was followed carefully and did well without antifungal therapy; a repeat chest computed tomography scan did not reveal any new pulmonary lesions that would be consistent with fungal infection.

Explanation and Consequences

Invasive aspergillosis occurs in a number of different clinical settings and continues to be associated with a high mortality rate [189]. Early diagnosis is critical to a favorable outcome, but is difficult to achieve with current diagnostic methods [190]. Deep tissue diagnostic specimens for histopathologic examination and fungal culture are ideal for diagnosing invasive aspergillosis and remain the gold standard; these specimens are often difficult to obtain from critically ill patients. Therefore, techniques in recent years have focused on the detection of circulating surrogate markers including genomic fungal DNA and fungal cell-wall components [191]. In particular, detection of circulating $(1 \rightarrow 3)$ β-glucan (galactomannan) has been a major advance in the diagnosis and management of invasive aspergillosis infections [192,193]. An important characteristic of the circulating galactomannan is that in approximately two-thirds of patients, this circulating antigen could be detected at a mean of 8 days before diagnosis by other means [192]. This characteristic has resulted in the circulating galactomannan test being used for prospective monitoring of patients during a period of high risk as was done in the previous case. However, reports of false-positive circulating galactomannan results caused by amoxicillin-clavulanic acid [187,194] and piperacillin-tazobactam [188,195] must be appreciated as they were in this case to avoid unnecessary use of antifungal therapy.

STANDARDS OF CARE

■ Failure to appreciate the sensitivity or specificity of microbiology tests can result in harm to a patient even though the correct diagnosis was considered, and an appropriate microbiology test was ordered; failure to appreciate the sensitivity or specificity of microbiology tests is a subtle but real form of medical error.

■ The sensitivity and specificity of antigen testing in clinical microbiology is particularly important; both false-negative and false-positive test results are factors in such antigen testing and must be appreciated.

■ Consultations with the clinical microbiology laboratory [127] and/ or the infectious diseases unit [128,129] are excellent ways to avoid this potential error.

FAILURE TO SUBMIT SUITABLE MICROBIOLOGY SPECIMEN

▶ Failure to submit suitable microbiology specimens is unfortunately a common problem that can lead to medical errors in infectious diseases and clinical microbiology. Consultation with the clinical microbiology laboratory regarding suitable specimens is the best way to avoid this error.

Case with Error

A healthy 29-year-old woman was seen in the emergency department with a chief complaint of a pustular and draining lesion on the lateral side of her right foot for 5 days. A nurse practitioner in another city had seen this patient 3 days earlier and had thought this abscess was caused by community-acquired methicillin-resistant *Staphylococcus aureus* (CA-MRSA). The nurse practitioner had performed an incision and drainage of the abscess and had also prescribed oral clindamycin; no cultures were done at this time. The abscess and cellulitis had worsened following the incision and drainage despite 3 days of oral clindamycin therapy, so the patient again sought medical assistance. Additional history obtained revealed that the patient had been on vacation in Mexico for several weeks prior to the onset of this pustular lesion; during this vacation, she had been water-cave exploring while barefoot. The physician seeing this patient in the emergency department was concerned that this infection might indeed be caused by CA-MRSA that was also resistant to clindamycin. Other water-borne microorganisms were considered as well. Therefore, the abscess was again incised and drained with purulent material sent for Gram stain and culture. The Gram stain revealed polymorphonuclear cells, but no organisms. There was initially no growth after several days of incubation, but the cultures were held because the clinician had alerted the microbiology laboratory that an unusual microorganism might be involved. On day 7, the cultures were positive for *Nocardia brasiliensis*. Because the patient was allergic to sulfa drugs, she was treated with oral minocycline for 6 months. The foot infection resolved on this therapy.

Explanation and Consequences

There are a number of areas of debate regarding management of skin and soft tissue abscesses [196]. These include the usefulness of cultures and empiric treatment with antimicrobial agents. In particular, the increasing incidence of CA-MRSA has intensified this debate. This case illustrates why there is a debate about cultures. The nurse practitioner that first saw this patient could justify not culturing this abscess based on the medical literature [196]. In fact, had a culture been done, it would have been negative at 48 hours and normally would not have been held longer than 48 hours. *Nocardia* species often take 5 days or longer to grow on sheep blood agar [197]. A "no growth" culture result would not have assisted in the care of this patient. However, the failure of the initial therapy prompted the elicitation of additional history as well as a culture to be held longer than 2 days; this allowed the diagnosis and appropriate therapy. Had this infection not been diagnosed, the *Nocardia* infection would have eventually involved deeper tissues and bone in the foot; this type of infection known as "Madura foot" is very difficult to treat and often leads to amputation of the infected foot [198].

Case with Error

This case [199] involves an 18-month-old boy who was admitted to a local hospital with a 4-day history of fever, cough, and increased respiratory rate. Physical examination revealed an alert child with a respiratory rate of 36 breaths per minute, a temperature of 105°F, and decreased breath sounds in the right lung. A chest radiograph showed infiltrates in the left lower lobe as well as in the right middle and right lower lobes; no pleural effusion was noted. Blood cultures and sputum cultures were not obtained. A presumptive diagnosis of community-acquired bacterial pneumonia was made, and the child was treated with intravenous cefuroxime for 3 days followed by oral cefuroxime for 2 days. The child remained febrile and thus received

an additional day of intravenous cefuroxime as well as a single dose
of intravenous ceftriaxone prior to discharge. The child was discharged home to complete a course of oral ceftibuten. However, the
child's fever persisted over the next 4 days, and the child was noted
to have an increased respiratory rate with grunting. The child therefore
was readmitted to the hospital. At this time, the respiratory rate was
76 with grunting, and the temperature was 102°F. A chest radiograph
revealed persistent infiltrates, but no pleural effusions. A lumbar puncture was done; this showed clear fluid with only 1 leukocyte/μL. The
cerebrospinal fluid was cultured. Blood cultures also were obtained.
The child was initially treated with intravenous vancomycin and
cefotaxime. A repeated chest radiograph showed a moderate pleural
effusion; a chest tube was inserted and 200 mL serosanguineous fluid
was drained. This fluid was not analyzed or cultured. The cerebrospinal fluid cultures were negative. However, the blood cultures were
positive for *Streptococcus pneumoniae*, which was resistant to beta-
lactam agents as well as to erythromycin. The child's fever resolved
on the fourth day of intravenous vancomycin and cefotaxime therapy;
the chest tube was removed at that time. Vancomycin and cefotaxime were continued for an additional 13 days. The child had a complete recovery.

Explanation and Consequences

The value of sputum Gram stain and culture in the diagnosis of
community-acquired pneumonia is another area in which there has
been considerable debate [200–205]. Moreover, obtaining a good-
quality sputum specimen is difficult in young, nonexpectorating
children with pneumonia [206]. Routine sputum collection and
analysis has not been recommended in children with community-
acquired pneumonia [207,208] for a number of reasons. Among
these cogent reasons are that viral pneumonia is the most common
cause of community-acquired pneumonia during the first 2 years and
that young children cannot easily expectorate sputum. Moreover,
empiric therapy with newer cephalosporins as done in this case generally has proven effective in situations in which clinicians suspect
a bacterial cause of community-acquired pneumonia in a child. As

illustrated in this case, resistance to newer cephalosporins can result in treatment failure leading to readmission to the hospital. A blood culture resulted in the etiologic agent in this case, and vancomycin therapy was responsible for the clinical success of the antimicrobial therapy used during the second admission. In this case, sputum cultures were not obtained on the second admission, although they could have been obtained using either induced sputum [209] or bronchoscopy [210]. Collection of sputum in children or in adults is likely to be very important in the near future when traditional diagnostic methods are supplemented with PCR-based methods in order to increase the microbiological yield for the etiology of community-acquired pneumonia [211].

Case with Error

This case [212] involves a 22-year-old man with chills and fever after a stay in South America. This young man was in excellent health and approximately 5 months earlier had enjoyed a 6-week trip to South America. This trip started in northern Ecuador with a prolonged stay in the jungle and included swimming in "dark waters" of lakes and rivers. The patient received many insect bites, consumed local food and fresh fruit, and remembers drinking water treated with an iodine filter. He experienced one episode of diarrhea for which he took three doses of ciprofloxacin. During the final 2 weeks of this trip, the patient traveled through the beaches and high mountains of Peru, hiked the Inca Trail, and visited Lima. The patient took doxycycline daily as prophylaxis and continued this for 2 weeks after returning. He was in his usual state of excellent health for almost 3 months following his trip to South America when he began to have a temperature as high as 40°C accompanied by chills, sweats, stiffness of his neck, and back pain. After several days of this fever, he went to the emergency room where his temperature was 40.1°C. Physical examination was essentially normal except for slight nuchal rigidity. A lumbar puncture was done and revealed clear, colorless cerebrospinal fluid that contained 2 RBCs and 0 WBCs/μL. A Gram stain revealed no microorganisms. The cerebrospinal fluid glucose and protein levels were normal. Blood cultures and cerebrospinal fluid cultures were done; these ultimately showed no growth. Other laboratory values included a normal complete blood count, normal electrolytes, and a normal creatinine. The patient was rehydrated with intravenous fluids and sent home from the emergency room with a diagnosis of "viral syndrome." Two days later, his fever returned; he again went to the emergency room where his temperature was 40.3°C. His physical examination at this time was unchanged. Repeat laboratory testing was unchanged except his platelet count had dropped from 128,000/μL to 92,000/μL. The results of the cultures done on the first emergency room visit were noted to be no growth; additional blood cultures were done. A chest radiograph was unremarkable. A mononucleosis test was negative. A throat culture was done; this ultimately was negative. The patient was rehydrated and sent home with a diagnosis of "viral syndrome." The patient continued to take acetaminophen and ibuprofen daily at home as this reduced the fever and chills. He was told to return for a follow-up visit in 1 week because of the thrombocytopenia. He did so, and on this follow-up visit 1 week later, his temperature was 36.8°C. He appeared slightly pale; his hematocrit was now 38% whereas it had been 43.2% only 1 week earlier. His bilirubin was noted to be slightly elevated at 1.3 mg/dL. The history of thrombocytopenia along with the decreased hematocrit and elevated bilirubin suggested the possibility of malaria; a blood sample was sent to the clinical microbiology laboratory for malaria evaluation. This allowed a diagnosis of *Plasmodium vivax* malaria infection to be made. The patient was successfully treated with both chloroquine and primaquine and has been well since.

Explanation and Consequences

This case nicely illustrates the failure to submit a suitable microbiology specimen, which in this instance would have been thin and thick smears for malaria evaluation. Although a complete blood count was done at each of the two emergency room visits, the peripheral blood examinations were performed using automated equipment. The number of fields scanned by a technologist on these smears using automated equipment is quite low and thus failure to pick up a light malarial parasitemia is not unusual [213]. More extensive scanning of the blood fields stored in automated blood equipment by a pathologist is, however, an excellent way to make a diagnosis of malaria. The first opportunity to diagnose malaria in this patient was the initial emergency room visit where the travel history to South America should have raised the possibility of malaria in the differential diagnosis. The key to the diagnosis of malaria is travel history as the incubation period can be variable for all strains of malaria. Indeed, fever in the returned traveler must always raise the possibility of malaria in the differential diagnosis [88,214–217]. In addition, imported malaria in visitors to the United States must also be considered in febrile patients with vague and nonspecific clinical presentations of malaria who may be seen in emergency rooms [89,218,219]. Thin and thick smears for malaria should be ordered as the parasitemia may be missed with routine complete blood counts done on automated instruments. The second opportunity to diagnose malaria in this patient was the secondary emergency room visit where the combination of travel to South America and thrombocytopenia should have prompted a blood smear evaluation for malaria. Thrombocytopenia is the most common laboratory abnormality encountered with malaria and is seen in approximately 60% of cases regardless of the type of malaria [220]. The diagnosis of malaria in this case was made on the third visit when the combination of travel to South America, thrombocytopenia, hyperbilirubinemia, and anemia were noted. Hyperbilirubinemia is seen in approximately 40% of malaria cases, and anemia is seen in approximately 30% [220]. The presence of thrombocytopenia and hyperbilirubinemia alone has a positive predictive value of 95% in the presumptive diagnosis of malaria in the febrile traveler returning from a part of the world where malaria is endemic [221]. It is important to understand that babesiosis can also present with fever, thrombocytopenia, hyperbilirubinemia, and anemia [82–84] and also may require thin and thick blood smears for diagnosis; routine complete blood counts on automated instruments may miss this diagnosis for the same reason as malaria can be missed [85,86,213]. Clearly, not sending blood for parasite analysis (i.e., malaria and babesiosis) can represent a failure to submit a suitable specimen in a febrile patient.

Case with Error

This case involves a 12-year-old previously healthy girl who jumped off a swing at school and landed on some wood chips. One of these wood chips penetrated her shoe and lodged deeply in her left heel. The child's grandmother, who was a nurse, removed the wood chip and cleaned the heel wound; this heel wound eventually closed. However, the child continued to have pain in her left heel when walking. After several months of this heel pain, a magnetic resonance imaging study of the left heel was done and revealed a calcaneal osteomyelitis. As *Staphylococcus aureus* is a common cause of calcaneal osteomyelitis in children [222], her local physician treated her with intravenous vancomycin via a PICC line for 2 months. No biopsy or culture was obtained. This empiric antimicrobial therapy did not resolve the left heel pain, and a bone biopsy was done 6 months after the original injury. A routine bacterial culture of this biopsy grew *Pantoea agglomerans,* which has been reported to cause infection after plant thorn and wood sliver injuries [223]. The child was treated for 6 weeks with oral sulfamethoxazole/trimethoprim base on susceptibility testing of the *P. agglomerans*; this therapy did not resolve the bone pain. Moreover, the biopsy site developed a violaceous lesion and would occasionally drain cloudy fluid. A repeat magnetic resonance imaging of the heel showed evidence of chronic osteomyelitis. Therefore, the child was referred to a pediatric orthopedic surgeon at a tertiary care center for a further evaluation. On admission, the child was afebrile. There was a 2 cm violaceous lesion located on the left heel at the site of a healed incision. The lesion was nontender; there was no erythema or induration surrounding this lesion. Laboratory values were normal and included a normal C-reactive protein and a normal erythrocyte sedimentation rate. The child was taken to the operating room for excision and debridement of the left heel osteomyelitis. In the process of scraping the inside of the bone cavity, two small wood fragments were retrieved; one measured 1 cm in length by 2 mm in width and the second was slightly smaller. Cultures for bacteria, fungi, and mycobacteria were ordered. After 2 weeks of incubation, the fungal cultures grew *Phialophora richardsiae.* The other cultures were negative. Susceptibility testing was done on this isolate of *P. richardsiae,* and it was susceptible to voriconazole. The child was successfully treated with oral voriconazole and has remained well.

Explanation and Consequences

This child was eventually diagnosed with chromoblastomycosis caused by *P. richardsiae*. Chromoblastomycosis is a chronic mycotic infection caused by pigmented saprophytic moulds of the Dermatiaceae family ubiquitous in the environment [224]. The members of the Dermatiaceae family are dimorphic filamentous fungi with melanic-type pigment in the cell wall. Clinically, the infection usually follows traumatic inoculation through penetrating thorn or splinter wounds and is characterized by the development of chronic verrucose lesions at the inoculation site. *P. richardsiae* is a recognized cause of chromoblastomycosis in humans [225,226] and can cause osteomyelitis [227]. There are a number of important points illustrated by this case. The first is that puncture wounds of the foot can result in serious complications such as osteomyelitis [228–230]. For this reason, puncture wounds may require wound enlargement and a search for a retained foreign body. Imbedded rubber foreign bodies [231] and thorn or wood splinters [226] are recognized risk factors for infection. A retained splinter of wood contributed to this child's prolonged infection. Another important point is that a biopsy with appropriate cultures should have been done initially rather than relying on empiric antimicrobial therapy with vancomycin. When cultures were done on this child, only routine bacterial cultures were ordered. It is possible that the *P. agglomerans* was a pathogen as gram-negative bacteria such as *Pseudomonas aeruginosa* can cause osteomyelitis following puncture wounds of the foot [230,232]. However, other microorganisms including fungi (as illustrated by this case) or mycobacteria [233] can also cause osteomyelitis of the calcaneus secondary to a puncture wound. It thus is important to realize that when cultures are ordered in calcaneal osteomyelitis following a puncture wound, bacterial, fungal, and mycobacterial cultures should be specified on the requisition.

Case with Error

This case (234) involves a 69-year-old woman who was admitted to an outlying hospital with fever and wrist pain. This woman had no other significant medical problems. On physical examination, the right wrist was tender with a decreased range of motion and an effusion. Laboratory values included a white blood cell count of 12,000/µL and an erythrocyte sedimentation rate of 34 mm/hour. A roentgenogram of the right wrist was unremarkable. Aspiration of the wrist yielded pus, which subsequently grew methicillin-susceptible *Staphylococcus aureus*. Therapy with intravenous oxacillin was initiated, and the patient seemed to respond. There were no stigmata of endocarditis noted. However, the patient developed pain in the thoracic area 1 week into the antimicrobial therapy, and over the next 24 hours also developed lower-extremity weakness. A chest radiograph was unremarkable. A computed tomography scan demonstrated a paravertebral abscess along T-8. This abscess was surgically drained and routine bacterial cultures were obtained; these cultures also grew *S. aureus*. Despite continued therapy with intravenous oxacillin, the patient worsened with continued fever, persistent leukocytosis, and the development of lower-extremity paralysis. Two months after admission, the patient was transferred to a tertiary care referral center for further evaluation. On admission to this referral center, the patient had a temperature of 39°C and appeared chronically ill with paraplegia. A careful evaluation for endocarditis was repeated and found no murmurs or peripheral stigmata of emboli. A repeat computed tomography scan of the spine revealed collapse of T-8 and a recurrent paraspinal abscess. This recurrent abscess was again surgically drained; this time, however, bone cultures were obtained for bacterial, fungal, and mycobacterial cultures. At 5 weeks, the mycobacterial cultures yielded *Mycobacterium tuberculosis*. Isoniazid and rifampin therapy was initiated for therapy of tuberculous osteomyelitis; the patient improved dramatically and eventually was discharged home albeit with residual paraplegia.

Explanation and Consequences

This case is another example of a mixed infection causing osteomyelitis. In this situation, *S. aureus* and *M. tuberculosis* were the microorganisms causing the osteomyelitis; similar cases can be found in the medical literature [235,236]. Had bone cultures for mycobacterium been done on the first hospital admission, this diagnosis might have been made earlier although it is unlikely that this paraplegia could have been avoided due to the length of time required for the growth of *M. tuberculosis*. If bone cultures for *Mycobacterium* are not done, and granulomatous inflammation without demonstrable acid-fast bacilli are seen, there are two potential solutions. The first solution is to recut the formalin-fixed, paraffin-embedded tissue for additional acid-fast staining. Additional sections cut for acid-fast staining will sometimes identify acid-fast bacilli not seen in the first cuts. The second solution is to use molecular detection methods such as PCR testing for *M. tuberculosis*; these are done on the formalin-fixed, paraffin-embedded tissue and have proven successful in such situations [237,238]. Such testing is best done in consultation with the clinical microbiology laboratory [127]. In general, bone specimens from patients with vertebral osteomyelitis should include bacterial, fungal, and mycobacterial cultures in order to avoid this type of medical error. Molecular testing is a reasonable adjunct test when mycobacterial cultures have not been done or are negative.

Case with Error

This case [238] involves an 18-year-old male of Somali origin who had been living in a Scandinavian country since the age of 7. The patient was referred to a hospital for recurrent bloody diarrhea, abdominal pain, fever, and weight loss. Physical examination was unremarkable except for abdominal distension and diffuse abdominal tenderness. A computed tomography scan of the chest and abdomen was unrevealing. A PPD skin test for tuberculosis was nonreactive. Colonoscopy revealed a segmental colitis with fissures; nodular and ulcerous lesions were also described along with a 10-cm stricture. Biopsies taken from these areas demonstrated discontinuous fissural submucosal inflammation; no granulomas were noted. Acid-fast staining of these tissue biopsies was negative for acid-fast bacilli; however, a gastric aspirate was positive by preliminary PCR testing for *M. tuberculosis*, thus therapy for tuberculosis was started. Conformational PCR testing of the gastric aspirate was negative and other cultures and PCR testing for *M. tuberculosis* from sputum, bronchial washings, gastric aspirates, stool, and blood were negative. After 1 week of therapy for tuberculosis without clinical improvement, this therapy was stopped. As the histology and endoscopic findings also were consistent with Crohn's disease, oral prednisone and intravenous nutrition were started. The patient seemed to respond to this approach, and the diarrhea ceased. Follow-up colonoscopy revealed decreased colitis, but three new fistulas were seen in the ascending colon. These fistulas were biopsied. Again, histopathologic stains revealed no acid-fast bacilli, and cultures for *M. tuberculosis* were negative; several noncaseating granuloma were seen in these biopsy specimens. Therapy for tuberculosis was restarted, and the steroid therapy was tapered. The patient was doing well and had gained weight when 2 months after admission he developed signs of an acute abdomen. An exploratory laparotomy was done and revealed small nodules throughout the peritoneal surfaces that suggested peritoneal tuberculosis. An ileocecal and ascending colon were done. Histology of the nodules, lymph nodes, and resected bowel segments demonstrated multiple caseating granulomas. Acid-fast stains were negative, but PCR assays of the granuloma were positive. The therapy for tuberculosis was continued, and the patient has done well.

Explanation and Consequences

The case illustrates the difficulty in diagnosing abdominal tuberculosis even when it is suspected [240–242]. Despite the multiple superficial biopsy specimens obtained by repeated colonoscopies as well as multiple other cultures and PCR assays obtained, none of these were diagnostic for gastrointestinal tuberculosis. Instead, a diagnosis of Crohn's disease was considered based on the noncaseating granuloma seen in biopsy specimens, and prednisone therapy was initiated. Endoscopic biopsy with histologic examination remains the best test for the initial diagnosis of Crohn's disease [243]. When tuberculosis is suspected, PCR for *M. tuberculosis* on biopsied tissue has been used to differentiate gastrointestinal tuberculosis from Crohn's disease [244] as was done in this case. The authors comment that the diagnosis of tuberculosis in this case might have occurred sooner if gastrointestinal lymph nodes had been biopsied [239]. The availability of laparoscopy for biopsy of gastrointestinal lymph nodes would suggest that when gastrointestinal tuberculosis is a possibility, laparoscopic biopsy of gastrointestinal lymph nodes should be considered due to the difficulty in making the diagnosis with more superficial biopsies done by endoscopy [245,246].

STANDARDS OF CARE

- Failure to submit a suitable microbiology specimen or any microbiology specimen at all even though infection is suspected may happen for a number of reasons and can be another subtle form of medical error.

- If unusual microorganisms are suspected, the clinical microbiology laboratory should be consulted as special media and/or incubating the cultures for a prolonged period of time might be necessary; such consultation [127] may also result in assistance in terms of what type of cultures should be ordered on specimens from a febrile patient.

- Consultation with infectious diseases [128,129] is also useful in determining what type of cultures should be obtained in a febrile patient.

- Fever in returning travelers or foreign travelers visiting the United States should raise the diagnostic possibility of malaria; thick and thin blood smears for malaria are indicated in this situation.

- Mixed infections with dissimilar microorganisms such as bacteria and fungi or bacteria and mycobacteria do occur; specimens sent to the clinical microbiology laboratory must specifically request bacterial, fungal, and mycobacterial cultures in order to ensure that all are done.

- Molecular diagnostic techniques now may offer a "second chance" to make the correct diagnosis if appropriate cultures are not requested on the specimen initially sent to the clinical microbiology laboratory.

- The pathophysiology of a suspected infection may provide insight on additional tissue that can be biopsied for culture and/or PCR testing when initial testing is nonrevealing.

FAILURE TO PROPERLY IDENTIFY PATIENT, SPECIMEN, OR TEST ORDER

> Failure to properly identify patient, specimen, or test order is a common issue in all laboratories. Attention to detail and electronic bar code labeling can assist with this problem.

Case with Averted Error

The clinical microbiology laboratory receives a set of blood culture bottles from the emergency room. These blood culture bottles have been inoculated with blood and are accompanied by a requisition for a blood culture. However, the blood culture bottles are not labeled with any patient information. The medical technologist then calls the emergency room and asks to speak to the nurse who obtained the blood culture and is taking care of this patient. This nurse is asked to come to the microbiology laboratory to properly label the blood culture bottles. The nurse complains that she is very busy and couldn't the medical technologist just label the blood culture bottles. After being told that this is against laboratory policy, the nurse reluctantly comes to the microbiology laboratory and labels the blood culture bottles. The nurse apologizes for not properly labeling the blood culture bottles initially, but states, "It is very busy in the emergency room, things are hectic, and I simply forgot to label the blood culture bottles."

Explanation and Consequences

This is an example of a patient misidentification error that was averted when detection of the unlabeled set of blood culture bottles by the microbiology technologist prompted a call to the emergency room so that the person who actually obtained the blood culture could come to the microbiology laboratory and properly label these bottles. Although rejection and recollection of a specimen once mislabeling is detected is the most suitable approach to managing this issue [247], this may not be possible for blood cultures if antimicrobial agents have been initiated. The unlabeled blood culture bottle might appear to be a minor issue that was easily resolved, but this type of preanalytic phase medical error is extremely common and has great potential for becoming a major issue. Assume that there could have been more than one unlabeled set of blood culture bottles, each set from two separate patients. Assume also that these were received in the microbiology laboratory at the same time. Properly labeling these two sets of blood culture bottles would become a major problem.

The preanalytic phase of laboratory testing is manually intense and thus prone to having the highest error rate [248]. Blood collection is a particularly error-prone portion of the total laboratory testing process. Among the common preanalytic phase errors are mistakes in tube filling, inappropriate containers, inappropriate requesting procedures, and identification errors (ie, misidentification). Indeed, misidentification has been identified as a major problem in the preanalytic phase of laboratory testing [249] with the following causes being the most problematic: (1) physician ordering a laboratory test on the wrong patient; (2) incorrect or incomplete computer entry of patient's data; (3) collection of a specimen from the wrong patient; (4) inappropriate labeling of the specimen; (5) lost identification (label or requisition) for the specimen; and (6) incorrect entry of the patient's results in the computer database.

Clearly the preanalytic phase of laboratory testing is vulnerable to errors; most of these errors result from system flaws and insufficient audit and control of the operators involved in specimen collection [248]. There are a number of factors that must be considered in order to deal with these types of preanalytic errors [250,251]. The first factor to consider is prediction of accidental events, which is accomplished by the following processes: (1) exhaustive process analysis; (2) reassessment and rearrangement of quality requirements; (3) dissemination of operating guidelines and best-practice recommendations; (4) reduction of complexity and error-prone activities; (5) introduction of error-tracking systems; (6) continuous monitoring of performance; and (7) root cause analysis of any errors identified to ensure that any systems flaws can be addressed. The next factor to consider is an increase in and diversification of defenses, which is accomplished by the application of multiple and heterogeneous systems to identify nonconformities. The final factor to consider is a decrease in vulnerability, which is accomplished by implementation of reliable and objective detection systems, causal relation charts, and education/training. These factors taken together constitute a systems approach for solving the problem of preanalytic errors.

STANDARDS OF CARE

■ The preanalytic phase of laboratory testing is manually intensive and prone to system flaws and operator error; a systems approach is required to avoid these kinds of errors.

■ Failure to properly identify a patient, specimen, or test order can be considered a "misidentification" error and is actually a common preanalytic error in laboratory testing that can result in minor inconvenience (eg, redrawing or relabeling) or in serious consequences (eg, wrong patient or delay in diagnosis); the "paperwork" must be considered an integral and important part of patient care.

■ Quality programs developed around the preanalytic phase of laboratory testing are required to avoid preanalytic errors; when errors occur, a root cause analysis must be done to identify any systems flaws that may contribute to such errors.

2

Analytic Errors in the Clinical Microbiology Laboratory

OVERVIEW

In contrast to preanalytic errors in laboratory testing, analytic errors have been carefully addressed in both the clinical microbiology laboratory [1,2,4] and in the laboratory as a whole [5,6]. Bartlett et al. [1] have comprehensively reviewed the process of managing quality in the clinical microbiology laboratory, and this review continues to serve as an ongoing template for a systems approach to quality. This does not mean that the analytic phase of testing in the clinical microbiology laboratory is error-free. Indeed, the detection and prevention of clinical microbiology laboratory-associated errors have been recognized and addressed by the American Society for Clinical Microbiology in their *Cumitech* series [252]. The *Cumitech* series is designed to provide consensus recommendations regarding the judicious use of clinical microbiology and immunology laboratories; each series is written by a team of clinicians, laboratorians, and other knowledgeable stakeholders to provide a broad overview of various important aspects of infectious diseases testing. The examples of analytic error that follow are selected from the medical literature as well as from the personal experience of the author and illustrate common medical errors within the clinical microbiology laboratory.

MISREADING OR MISINTERPRETATION OF GRAM STAIN OR OTHER STAINS

▶ Misreading or misinterpretation of Gram stain or other stains is not a common problem in most clinical microbiology laboratories, but does occasionally happen. There are technical issues that usually contribute to this problem when it happens. These technical issues should be understood.

Case with Error

This case [253] involves a 42-year-old man who was being evaluated for fever and a stiff neck. His first lumbar puncture demonstrated 80 lymphocytes/mL in the cerebrospinal fluid; the Gram stain and culture of this fluid were unrevealing. The patient spontaneously improved, but 2 weeks later had a recurrence of his fever and stiff neck. The lumbar puncture was repeated; cerebrospinal fluid analysis revealed a leukocyte count of 940 cells/µL with 50% polymorphonuclear cells. The cerebrospinal fluid glucose level was low, and the protein level was elevated. The Gram stain was read as many small gram-negative cocci, and the patient was treated for *Neisseria* meningitis. Despite this antimicrobial therapy for meningococcal meningitis, the patient's condition worsened. All bacterial cultures had no growth. The lumbar puncture was repeated a third time; the Gram stain was unrevealing. However, an India ink preparation done for the first time revealed encapsulated budding yeast. Culture of the cerebrospinal fluid grew *Cryptococcus neoformans*. The patient expired; autopsy findings showed disseminated cryptococcosis with no evidence of bacterial infection.

Explanation and Consequences

This case illustrates the well-recognized difficulty of diagnosing cryptococcal meningitis [178,254]. In this particular case, a misread Gram stain of the cerebrospinal fluid contributed to the initial diagnostic confusion. In general, the microscopic examination of cerebrospinal fluid in the diagnosis of meningitis is quite sensitive ranging from 67% to 92% [255,256]. It is rare for cerebrospinal fluid examinations to incorrectly suggest the presence of microorganisms. *C. neoformans* is known to be confusing on Gram stain with both gram-positive and gram-negative misidentification being reported [257]. A high index of suspicion for cryptococcal meningitis along with the use of the cryptococcal antigen test [177] is a key factor in the diagnosis of such meningitis and will help avoid delays in treatment.

Clearly the rapid and accurate detection and characterization of microorganisms encountered in purulent cerebrospinal fluid from patients with meningitis is important [255,256,258]. Misreading a Gram stain from a cerebrospinal fluid specimen is unusual, but can happen [253]. There are a number of ways to avoid such misreading errors. Quality assessment programs in the clinical microbiology laboratory [1,2] include both internal and external proficiency testing as well as the testing of microbiology technologists for color-blindness. Such competency assessment in the clinical microbiology laboratory [259] is an important, ongoing function that prevents such errors [252]. In addition, most clinical microbiology laboratories routinely have a senior microbiologist review any positive Gram stains from cerebrospinal fluid. Finally, other causes of false-positive Gram stains from cerebrospinal fluid not infrequently have been described [260–265] and are not due to misreading the Gram stain. Instead, contamination with nonviable bacteria from various products used in the process is the cause of such false-positive Gram stains of cerebrospinal fluid. This issue will be discussed in greater detail in the next case.

Case with Error

This series of cases [264] begins with a febrile patient with neurologic symptoms whose cerebrospinal fluid obtained by lumbar puncture demonstrated gram-negative bacilli on smears. This patient was treated with cefotaxime for 3 days before a diagnosis of carcinomatous meningitis was made. All cultures were negative for any growth. The antimicrobial therapy was discontinued without adverse consequences. Over the next week, three more cerebrospinal fluid specimens from three additional patients revealed gram-negative bacilli that failed to grow in any cultures. This cluster of nonviable gram-negative bacilli that were seen on cerebrospinal fluid Gram stains lead to an investigation of the lumbar puncture trays. The results of this investigation revealed that specimen tubes in these lumbar puncture trays were contaminated with nonviable gram-negative bacilli. A further investigation by the FDA revealed that almost one-quarter of the specimen tubes from commercial lumbar puncture trays contained nonviable gram-negative bacilli with numbers of bacilli per tube ranging from 44 to 332.

Explanation and Consequences

The Gram stain of cerebrospinal fluid is recognized as critical in the diagnostic evaluation of a patient with suspected meningitis, and positive Gram stains revealing microorganisms are used to direct initial therapy [3]. Clinicians and laboratory personnel usually do not consider a false-positive Gram stain from cerebrospinal fluid to be a potential problem. However, it must be appreciated that such false-positive Gram stains can occur. Factitious meningitis due to nonviable bacteria in commercial lumbar puncture trays was first reported in the mid-1970s and has continued to be seen [260–265]. The medical products industry has effectively ensured the sterility of commercial medical devices, but the procedures used to sterilize these products do not prevent the presence of nonviable microorganisms. Therefore, physicians and laboratory personnel must be aware that such false-positive Gram stains may occur. Although specimen tubes in lumbar puncture trays are the most common cause of factitious meningitis, other sources of nonviable microorganisms such as cytocentrifuge funnels and Gram-stain reagents may be a source [262,265]. The laboratory must review any specimen showing microorganisms on direct smears that fail to grow. If factitious organisms are suspected, the physician should be notified. If possible, a repeat cerebrospinal fluid specimen should be obtained using new, clean sterile glass tubes. Any cluster of such cases should be reported to the FDA.

Case with Error

This case [266] involves a previously healthy 14-month-old boy who was initially seen for fever, irritability, and vomiting. The child had been febrile for 2 days before being brought to a pediatric outpatient clinic. The child's mother said her son had also been vomiting and was irritable. On physical examination, the boy was noted to have a stiff neck and therefore was admitted to the hospital. Initial laboratory values included a white blood cell count of 13,800/μL with 71% neutrophils. A lumbar puncture done on admission revealed a cerebrospinal fluid cell count of 101 cells/μL, a cerebrospinal fluid protein level of 215 mg/dL, and a cerebrospinal fluid glucose level of 9 mg/dL. The cerebrospinal fluid Gram stain demonstrated gram-positive diplococcus-like microorganisms that were thought to be *Streptococcus pneumoniae*. A diagnosis of bacterial meningitis was made, and the child was treated with a combination of ceftriaxone and panipenem. The cerebrospinal fluid culture grew *Acinetobacter baumannii*. The patient's antimicrobial therapy was changed to meropenem based on susceptibility testing results. The child recovered with no central nervous system sequelae.

Explanation and Consequences

This child presented with community-acquired meningitis, and *S. pneumoniae* is a common cause of community-acquired meningitis in pediatric patients. Thus, the interpretation of the cerebrospinal fluid Gram stain was reasonable. The cerebrospinal fluid culture grew *A. baumannii*, which is a short, plump, gram-negative rod that is difficult to destain and may therefore be misidentified as a gram-positive diplococcus [267]. Fortunately, the broad-spectrum antimicrobial therapy used in this case provided coverage against this patient's isolate. *A. baumannii* rarely causes community-acquired meningitis, although it has been reported as a cause of community-acquired pneumonia [268]. This child had no evidence of pneumonia. When *A. baumannii* is seen as a cause of meningitis in a child, it usually follows a neurosurgical procedure and is multidrug-resistant [269]. Fortunately, this child's isolate was not multidrug-resistant.

Case with Error

A healthy 36-year-old man involved in a motor vehicle accident was admitted to the trauma unit with a high-energy, open fracture of the lower third of his right tibia. There was no evidence of crush injury to the limb, and the patient was hemodynamically stable. No other injuries were detected. The patient was taken to surgery for debridement, open reduction, and internal fixation. The patient did well following this surgery until postoperative day 3 when the surgical wound site became inflamed, swollen, and extremely tender, with an associated elevation in his white blood cell count and an elevated C-reactive protein. Infection was suspected, and empiric antimicrobial therapy with intravenous imipenem was initiated. The patient was taken to the operating room for exploration of the operative site as well as debridement, drainage, and cultures if indicated. The operative site was found to have a small amount of tissue necrosis as well as purulent material; there was no widespread tissue necrosis noted. Debridement was done, and necrotic tissue and purulent material were sent for cultures. The Gram-stain smear for this purulent material was read as gram-negative bacilli. However, the culture result on the following day was *Bacillus cereus*, which was susceptible to imipenem. The patient was continued on the imipenem and recovered without further problems.

Explanation and Consequences

This case illustrates an issue with the Gram stain that is well known to microbiologists but not to physicians, which is Gram-stain variability in select bacteria including *Bacillus* species [270]. *B. cereus* was isolated from the trauma-related orthopedic wound infection in this patient; such *Bacillus* infections have been reported in orthopedic trauma cases [271]. *Bacillus* species including *B. cereus* is known to be gram-variable and can stain as gram-negative bacilli as well as gram-positive filamentous forms that show beading and be confused with *Nocardia* species [270–273]. In this case, the isolate was susceptible to imipenem. This was fortunate as *B. cereus* produces multiple beta-lactamases, which include a metallo-beta-lactamase. These beta-lactamases are very potent against beta-lactam agents, including the third-generation cephalosporins. Imipenem and other carbapenem agents seem to be active against *B. cereus* despite the presence of this metallo-beta-lactamase [272,273]. However, carbapenem-resistant strains of *B. cereus* have been reported [274]. Vancomycin or clindamycin are preferred choices for therapy of *B. cereus* infections.

Case with Averted Error

This case [275] involves a 9-year-old boy who was acutely hospitalized because of a 43% full thickness, 53% total body surface burn. The patient was treated with fluid resuscitation and had multiple escharotomies and graft placements during the first 2 weeks of hospitalization. The child did well until hospital day 17 when he developed fever, leukocytosis with a left shift, and an elevated C-reactive protein. After cultures were obtained, the boy was treated with empirical antimicrobial therapy consisting of piperacillin/tazobactam and vancomycin. Blood, peritoneal fluid, tracheal aspirate, and graft cultures subsequently grew *Serratia marcescens*, which was susceptible to the piperacillin/tazobactam. The child's clinical condition initially worsened due to the sepsis, and he developed metabolic acidosis and acute renal failure. However, he stabilized and then gradually improved with the antimicrobial therapy. On day 4 of antimicrobial therapy, repeat blood cultures were done. The Gram stain from these blood cultures revealed long, filamentous gram-negative rods with hyphal-like characteristics. Subcultures of these blood cultures revealed gram-negative bacilli. The microbiology technologist noted the morphologic differences between the Gram-stain smears from the blood culture bottles and the microorganisms growing from subcultures. A second fungal pathogen was considered. Because the child was improving when the blood cultures were done, fungal therapy was not initiated. The final blood culture revealed only *S. marcescens*. The patient was continue on the same antimicrobial therapy and improved without additional complications. On postburn day 66, the child was transferred to the rehabilitation unit for physical therapy.

Explanation and Consequences

This case illustrates morphologic changes that can be seen in gram-negative bacilli that are exposed to certain beta-lactam agents. In this case, the piperacillin interacting with penicillin-binding proteins results in cell elongation without division [276]. These filamentous forms may appear by Gram stain to be a fungal pathogen. Because the child was improving, antifungal therapy was not initiated. However, it can easily be appreciated that such antifungal therapy might have been added if the child had not been improving.

This case also illustrates misinterpretation of a Gram stain from a positive blood culture. Prompt Gram staining of positive blood cultures is recognized as an important factor in directing antimicrobial therapy and has been shown to decrease mortality [277]. As mentioned earlier, physicians rarely question the accuracy of such Gram stains. Yet, the exigencies of the staining properties of certain species of bacteria [270] as well as human interpretive error can result in misinterpretation of a Gram stain from a positive blood culture. Indeed, misinterpretation of Gram stains from positive blood cultures has been reported for certain species of bacteria as well as for instances of underdecolorization or overdecolorazation of the Gram stain [278,279]. In this report, two systematic errors were noted. In 11 cases, *Bacillus* species were read as gram-negative bacilli; this is known to be a problem with this species [270]. In 5 cases, *Acinetobacter* species were read as gram-positive cocci or gram-positive bacilli; this is also known to be a problem with this species [267].

Underdecolorization and overdecolorization of the Gram stain is related to the use of acetone and isopropanol in the decolorization step.

Acetone is too strong a decolorizer for gram-positive microorganisms while isopropanol is too weak a decolorizer for gram-negative microorganisms. Therefore, most Gram-stain kits use a mixture of one part acetone to three parts of isopropanol. The decolorization step should be done until the solvent running from the slide is colorless. Safranin or fuchsin are used as a counterstain and should be applied for 30 to 60 seconds. Prolonged application may cause gram-positive microorganisms to appear gram negative, while short application may cause gram-negative microorganisms to appear gram positive. The timing and the acetone/isopropanol ratio as well as the species of microorganism all are important factors in the Gram stain. For Gram stains of clinical specimens that include polymorphonuclear cells in the background, a good quality control indicator is that occasionally the nucleus of a polymorphonuclear cell should stain purple. If most of the nuclei are staining purple, the stain is underdecolorized. If no purple nuclei can be seen after reviewing multiple fields, the stain is overdecolorized. If a Gram stain is considered underdecolorized or overdecolorized, the slide can be washed with xylene and the stain repeated.

Clearly, the answer to the question, "Can we always trust the Gram stain?" [279] is "No." Misread Gram stains from positive blood cultures are generally recognized within 1 to 2 days when the microorganism grown on plates is recognized as being inconsistent with the Gram-stain report; an amended report should be done. In addition, the physician should be notified by telephone.

Case with Averted Error

A 35-year-old woman developed an enlarging, tender nodule on the dorsal aspect of her right ankle. This nodule was located in a newly healed burn scar; the burn had occurred 4 months earlier when she had burned her ankle on a hot motorcycle exhaust. The nodule had grown rapidly over the past month and thus was completely excised. The histopathologic examination of the hematoxylin and eosin (H&E) slides revealed a dermal lesion with invagination of the epidermis and a central crater that was filled with eosinophilic keratinous material. These findings were consistent with the diagnosis of keratoacanthoma, which has been reported as arising in burn scars [280]. However, the

H&E stain also revealed brown septate hypal structures that raised the question of chromoblastomycosis [281] although no similar fungal forms were seen in the Gomori-methenamine silver (GMS) stain. A clinical microbiologist was asked to review the H&E and GMS slides and noted that there was minimal inflammation associated with this lesion; fungal contamination during slide preparation was therefore suspected as the source of the hypal structures seen on the H&E stain. The H&E stain reagents were replaced, and the H&E stain repeated; no fungal elements were seen on the repeated H&E slide.

Explanation and Consequences

This case illustrates one of the problems that artifacts and organism mimickers can pose in the diagnosis of infection [282]. Of these problem, fungal elements from contamination during slide preparation is the most difficult to deal with because these will stain with GMS and PAS stains. Pathologists and microbiologist need to assess the tissue inflammatory response when fungal elements are seen; if the cellular response is inconsistent, fungal contamination during slide preparation must be considered.

An additional mimicker of fungal yeast elements can be seen in H&E stains from dermal lesions in which there is inflammation and plasma cells. This mimic is Russell bodies, which are intracytoplasmic immunoglobulin bodies in plasma cells [283]. Russell bodies have been reported to cause confusion with blastomycosis [284] as well as other pathogenic fungi such as *Histoplasma, Cryptococcus*, and *Candida* species that have yeast forms [285]. Russell bodies are of variable size and lack the budding characteristics of these pathogenic fungi. Although Russell bodies are positive with PAS stains, they stain brown-gray with GMS, not black as would be expected.

Case with Error

A 17-year-old boy was admitted to a children's hospital because of a several-week history of pain and swelling in his right elbow following an injury to this elbow. An initial radiograph of the elbow taken soon after the elbow injury had been unremarkable, but a second radiograph done 2 weeks later revealed evidence of osteomyelitis. Examination of the elbow revealed a decreased range of motion, point tenderness over the proximal ulna, and signs of an effusion over the humeroulnar joint. Laboratory studies included a white blood cell count of 11,000 cells/μL, a C-reactive protein of 47.4 mg/L, and an ESR of 88 mm/hour. A magnetic resonance imaging (MRI) study showed chronic osteomyelitis of the proximal ulna as well as an exuberant mass surrounding the lesion that was thought to be granulation tissue, but a sarcoma could not be ruled out. Given the severity of the MRI report, an open biopsy was done and an intraoperative frozen section of the proximal ulna bone was sent to surgical pathology because the surgeon was concerned about the possibility of a sarcoma [286,287]. The slides evaluated from the frozen section did not show sarcoma, but instead revealed a fungal osteomyelitis with only a few fungal microorganisms being seen. These fungal microorganisms were large yeastlike structures with no budding suggesting a young spherule; a refractile cell wall was not seen. Unfortunately, at the time of the frozen section evaluation, a travel history was not provided to the pathologist. The morphological findings were reported as fungal osteomyelitis with *Coccidioides* being favored. The subsequent Gomori-methenamine silver (GMS) and periodic acid-Schiff (PAS) stains from permanent sections revealed yeast forms with broad-based budding and a thick refractive cell wall. These microscopic finding suggested *Blastomyces dermatitidis*; cultures obtained as surgery confirmed this diagnosis. The patient was treated with oral itraconazole and has done well.

Explanation and Consequences

This case illustrates the difficulty of evaluating frozen sections [288]. Although the frozen section evaluation in this case was able to correctly identify a fungal osteomyelitis, it was not able to identify the specific fungal pathogen causing the osteomyelitis. The differential for fungal osteomyelitis in this case included blastomycosis [289], cryptococcosis [290], and coccidioidomycosis [291]. Even with special GMS or PAS stains, identifying a specific fungal microorganism from tissue may be difficult even for experienced pathologists and microbiologists [292,293]. A 10-year retrospective study at Stanford University Medical Center found that 79% of fungal organisms with concurrent positive cultures were correctly identified based on morphologic characteristics by surgical pathology evaluation [293]. Common errors found in this study included morphologic mimics, poor sampling of tissue, use of inappropriate terminology, and lack of knowledge with regard to mycology. Morphologic identification can be a useful tool for the preliminary diagnosis of fungal infection, but culture remains the gold standard for speciation. All should be used concurrently to ensure that an accurate diagnosis is made. In this case, lack of budding in the frozen section stain made *B. dermatitidis* difficult to distinguish from *Coccidioides*. Moreover, empty, overlapping spherules in *Coccidioides* can mimic budding yeast and be mistaken for *B. dermatitidis* broad-based yeast in the process of budding [293]. The Alcian blue or an acid-fast stain can be used to distinguish between *Coccidioides* and *Blastomyces*; *Coccidioides* is negative and *Blastomyces* is weakly positive. Some recommend the presence of at least one intact spherule containing endospores before making a diagnosis of *Coccidioides* in tissue [293]. Other special stains can be used to distinguish *Blastomyces* from *Cryptococcus*. Cryptococcus usually will stain strongly with mucicarmine; the occasional capsule-deficient forms of cryptococci stain with melanin [295]. In contrast, the cell wall of *Blastomyces* is only weakly positive when stained with mucicarmine and negative with melanin. In this case, the GMS stains readily allowed the diagnosis of blastomycosis to be made.

STANDARDS OF CARE

■ Gram stains or other stains can be misread and/or misinterpreted due to a number of technical reasons; these reasons are understood by clinical microbiologists and pathologists, but may not be understood by physicians taking care of the patient.

■ When misreading and/or misinterpreting as stain occurs and is recognized, a corrected report must be entered into the health record; moreover, the clinicians involved should be called and told of this error.

■ A root cause analysis should be done for misreading and/or misinterpreting a stain in order to determine if there are any recurring systems issues that can be corrected.

■ Because many errors caused by misreading and/or misinterpreting a stain cannot be completely avoided due to technical reasons, it is important that microbiologists/pathologists maintain clear communication channels with clinicians in order to quickly resolve and correct such errors when they occur.

MISIDENTIFICATION OF MICROORGANISM

> ▶ Misidentification of a microorganism does not occur frequently, but can happen. Often there are technical issues that must be appreciated. Correction of the misidentification in the medical record and timely communication of the misidentification is important.

Case with Error

This case [296] is that of a previously healthy 35-year-old man who was admitted to a hospital in Switzerland because of an extradural cranial abscess of the right parietal area with a defect in the adjacent bone. This man had recently traveled to Singapore, Malaysia, and Thailand, but did not remember receiving a head injury during his trip. Approximately 2 weeks after returning from this trip, the patient noticed a swelling in the right parietal area that was gradually increasing in size; attempted aspiration of this bulge produced no aspirate. Over the next 2 months, the parietal bulge became painful, and secretion of pus was noted at the time of admission. On admission, the patient was in no distress and had no signs of systemic inflammation. Physical examination revealed no neurologic deficits; the only abnormal finding was the parietal bulge. Laboratory tests included a complete blood cell count and a C-reactive protein; test results were normal. A computed tomography scan and magnetic resonance imaging of the head showed an abscess and a small defect of bone in the right parietal area. The abscess and part of the parietal bone were surgically removed. Cultures of the abscess and bone biopsy specimens grew smooth creamy colonies on sheep blood agar; these colonies yielded gram-negative, oxidase-positive bacilli. For identification, the isolate was tested using the UNMIC/ID-62 panel of the BD Phoenix Automated Microbiology System [297]. This system identified the isolate as *Burkholderia cepacia* (99% confidence). The patient was discharged from the hospital with a tentative diagnosis of *B. cepacia* infection of soft tissue; the bone lesion was attributed to trauma. The patient was treated for 16 days with sulfamethoxazole/trimethoprim to which the isolate was susceptible. However, subsequent molecular verification of this isolate revealed that it was *Burkholderia pseudomallei*. The patient was readmitted to the hospital 44 days after surgery, and new biopsy specimens were collected and cultured for *B. pseudomallei*; these cultures were negative. Despite these negative cultures, 2 weeks of oral sulfamethoxizole/trimethoprim that the patient had received was considered inadequate. To ensure complete eradication of *B. pseudomallei*, the patient was treated with intravenous imipenem and sulfamethoxazole/trimethoprim for 2 weeks followed by oral therapy with sulfamethoxazole/trimethoprim for 6 months. After completing this therapy, there was only a small indentation in the parietal bone and no signs of inflammation.

Explanation and Consequences

The initial diagnosis of *B. cepacia* infection in this case was suspect to the microbiologist involved for a number of reasons, which included an unexpected, earthy odor of the bacterial colonies, unexpected susceptibility to amoxicillin/clavulanate, and an unexpected location and type of infection for a presumed *B. cepacia* abscess. In addition, automated identification systems are known for misidentification of isolates of the *Burkholderia cepacia* complex (BCC), and molecular methods for confirmatory identification of BCC are highly recommended [298]. Accordingly, the isolate from this case was verified by amplification and sequencing a 500-bp fragment of the 16S rRNA gene; these results suggested that the isolate was *B. pseudomallei*.

B. pseudomallei is the cause of melioidosis, a serious infection common in Southwest Asia [299,300]. This result thus raised two areas of concern. The first was the therapy of the patient. The patient had been treated with 2 weeks of sulfamethoxazole/trimethoprim, which would not be considered adequate therapy for an abscess/osteomyelitis caused by *B. pseudomallei*. In fact, treatment of any infection caused by *B. pseudomallei* is difficult, and there is a high rate of relapse if prolonged therapy is not completed. Generally 2 weeks of intravenous therapy with ceftazidime or a carbapenem is given followed by at least 4 months of oral sulfamethoxizole/trimethoprim. The second issue raised was the safety of laboratory personnel exposed to this pathogen [301]. Fortunately, the exposure to laboratory personnel in this case was classified as a low risk; no personnel became ill or showed signs of melioidosis.

Automated systems for identification and antimicrobial susceptibility testing of bacterial isolates, such as the Phoenix System, have become standard in most clinical laboratories. Identification of bacterial isolates is dependent on the database of the automated system; *B. pseudomallei* was not in the database of the Phoenix System. Currently, the most rapid and accurate identification method for *B. pseudomallei* is a manual method that uses the API 20NE system combined with a noncommercial latex agglutination test [302]. Molecular methods are accurate, but take more time. However, the clinical presentation in this case argued against this isolate being a *B. cepacia*, and verification was done. This resulted in the correct diagnosis. The limitations of automated systems must be understood by clinical microbiologists in order to avoid this type of identification error.

Case with Averted Error

A 25-year-old male graduate student is seen in July at a university student health clinic with a chief complaint of sore throat accompanied by fever, chills, and night sweats. The young man had been sick for 3 days with malaise, fatigue, sore throat, fever, chills, and night sweats. His past medical history was unremarkable. Physical examination revealed tonsilar enlargement with exudate and enlarged, tender posterior cervical lymph nodes. During his visit, a rapid antigen test for group A streptococci was done and was negative. A mononucleosis spot test also was done and was positive. A diagnosis of mononucleosis was made. The patient was treated with 6 days of methylprednisolone given in a decreasing dose along with an analgesic mouthwash for symptomatic relief. A week later, the student returned to the student health clinic because he was not getting better. Laboratory tests at this time revealed elevated liver enzymes, thrombocytopenia, and an elevated white blood cell count. A diagnosis of mild hepatitis related to his mononucleosis was made, and the patient was again sent home. He returns within a day because of fever, weakness, and feeling lightheaded when he stood. At this time, he was noted to have tachycardia and was hypotensive; therefore, he was referred to the emergency room. In the emergency room, his temperature is 101°F, his pulse is 134 bpm, and his blood pressure is 88/64 mm Hg while standing. Laboratory tests included a white blood cell count of 19,100/µL with 91% neutrophils, a platelet count of 45,000/µL, and mildly elevated liver function studies. The patient was admitted for possible ehrlichiosis and doxycycline was started. Blood cultures drawn in the emergency room were positive within 24 hours for a beta-hemolytic streptococcus that was identified by the Phoenix Automated Microbiology System as a group C streptococcus [303]. The clinical microbiologist considered this identification to be unlikely; group C streptococcus can cause severe acute pharyngitis in young adults [304] but is rarely isolated from blood cultures [305]. The clinical microbiologist also noted a caramel odor [306,307] on the isolation plate and thus considered *Streptococcus constellatus* subspecies *pharyngitis* to be a more likely cause of the bacteremia in this patient as this microorganism is known to be beta-hemolytic, can produce diacetyl (caramel odor) and can cross-react with Lancefield group C antigens [306–309]. Meanwhile, a chest roentgenogram revealed multiple cavitary lesions; septic emboli from endocarditis were considered based on the positive blood culture and the cavitary pulmonary lesions. Intravenous cefepime and levofloxacin were started. A transthoracic echocardiogram was done and did not reveal any vegetations. A review of the electronic health record by the clinical microbiologist in which the cavitary pulmonary lesions were noted led to consideration of Lemierre's syndrome. Physicians taking care of the patient agreed with this possibility, and a bilateral internal jugular venous ultrasound was done. The ultrasound revealed a thrombus in his right internal jugular vein, and a diagnosis of Lemierre's syndrome was made. The patient was treated with intraveneous ceftriaxone and heparin. Although prolonged hospitalization for this treatment was required, the patient eventually recovered completely and was discharged.

Explanation and Consequences

This case illustrates three important points. The first is a medical error caused by misidentification of a microorganism. Although in this case, the Phoenix Automated Microbiology System was responsible for this error, other identification methods are known to have difficulty distinguishing *S. constellatus* and other members of the *S. anginosus* (aka *S. milleri*) group from group C streptococci (*S. equisimilis*) [309]. Many clinical microbiology laboratories presumptively identify beta-hemolytic streptococci on the basis of Lancefield grouping. Some of the group C streptococcal bacteremia cases reported in the medical literature [305] may actually represent bacteremia by members of the *S. anginosus* group [309]. Differentiation of group C streptococci from members of the *S. anginosus* group is best accomplished by the Voges-Proskauer (VP) test [310]; members of the *S. anginosus* group produce acetoin whereas *S. equisimilis* does not. In this case, the Phoenix Automated Microbiology System cannot be expected to detect diacetyl (caramel odor); moreover, the Phoenix Streptococcal Panel does not include the VP test.

The second point illustrated by this case is that isolation of a member of the *S. anginosus* group from a blood culture is a "sentinel result" [7], because these pathogens can be associated with abscesses and/or suppurative thrombophlebitis [311,312]. It is important that clinical microbiologists appreciate the potential pathogenicity of *S. anginosus* isolates and alert clinicians to this potential pathogenicity. This type of sentinel result has been termed a "vital value" [313]; alerting clinicians of such a result can promote patient safety by preventing a medical error [314] and is an example of "enhanced clinical consulting" [315]. In this case, the availability of an electronic health record [316] allowed a review of the clinical information on this patient and facilitated the diagnosis of Lemierre's syndrome [317].

The third point illustrated by this case is the difficulty that can be seen with the diagnosis of Lemierre's syndrome. This suppurative thrombophlebitis of the internal jugular vein often involves septic emboli and metastatic infection [317–319]. Severe complications and death may occur when the diagnosis of Lemierre's syndrome is unsuspected or delayed. The clinical presentation of Lemierre's syndrome typically involves a young, previously healthy person who initially has a sore throat and subsequently develops persistent high fever. One half of the patients will present with ipsilateral neck pain and swelling; tenderness, trismus, or a thrombosied jugular vein may be found on physical examination of the neck. Metastatic abscesses are often seen; these abscesses may involve the lung and result in cavitary pulmonary lesions that can be seen on a chest radiograph. The main pathogen is *Fusobacterium necrophorum*, which is a common but unappreciated cause of pharyngitis in adolescents and young adults [320]. In addition, members of the *S. anginosus* group can cause Lemierre's syndrome [321]. Often the diagnosis of Lemierre's syndrome is first suggested when *F. necrophorum* or a member of the *S. anginosus* group is isolated from a blood culture. Clinical microbiologists have a key role in alerting clinicians to the possibility of Lemierre's syndrome when these microorganisms are isolated from blood cultures. Contrast-enhanced computed tomography scan of the neck can confirm the diagnosis of suppurative thrombophlebitis of the internal jugular vein.

Case with Error

This case [322] involves a 29-year-old woman with end-stage renal disease requiring dialysis who was admitted to the hospital with a 3-week history of fatigue and weakness. She was status post two failed kidney transplants and had a previous infection of her dialysis catheter that was left in place and treated with antibiotics. Physical examination revealed an elevated temperature of 37.9°C as well as a grade 2 systolic ejection murmur heard best in the right upper sternal border. A transesophageal echocardiogram demonstrated large vegetations on the anterior mitral valve leaflet. Blood cultures were positive for an aerobic non-spore-forming gram-positive bacillus that was reported as *Corynebacterium* spp. Further identification was done using the Crystal Gram Positive Rods System (BBL), the microorganism was identified as *Corynebacterium pseudogenitalium*, but only with 68% confidence. Susceptibility testing was done using the E-test; the microorganism was susceptible to vancomycin, penicillin, gentamicin, clindamycin, and ceftriaxone. Antimicrobial therapy was initiated with intermittent vancomycin dosed with hemodialysis sessions. Despite this antimicrobial therapy, blood cultures continued to grow *Corynebacterium*. On day 10 of vancomycin therapy the patient became septic. Blood cultures again grew *Corynebacterium*; a repeat echocardiogram revealed persistence of vegetations. Her antimicrobial therapy was broadened empirically with the addition of gentamicin and piperacillin-tazobactam. Her sepsis began to resolve, and her blood cultures became sterile. However, 10 days later her condition again deteriorated, and blood cultures were again positive for *Corynebacterium*. An acid-fast stain was done at this time and was positive; this allowed the microorganism to be identified as *Mycobacterium abscessus* Imipenem, clarithromycin, and moxifloxacin were initiated empirically; susceptibility testing at a reference laboratory revealed a very resistant strain. While on therapy, the patient unfortunately developed complications of her hospitalization, including candidemia and hospital-acquired pneumonia. These complications resulted in the patient's demise 24 days after initiation of therapy.

Explanation and Consequences

In this case, misidentification of *M. abscessus* resulted in a substantial delay in the administration of optimal antimicrobial therapy against this pathogen. *M. abscessus* is a member of the rapidly growing mycobacteria [323]; these rapidly growing mycobacteria are unusual causes of endocarditis [324,325]. Rapidly growing mycobacteria can easily be misidentified as *Nocardia* spp. or *Corynebacterium* spp. This potential for misidentification is illustrated by a European quality control report [326] in *M. fortuitum* specimens labeled as "pus from an abscess" were sent to 50 clinical microbiology laboratories for proficiency testing. Only 13 of the 50 laboratories correctly identified *M. fortuitum*. These specimens were misidentified as *Nocardia* spp. (23 laboratories) or *Corynebacterium* spp. (14 laboratories). Indeed, misidentification of rapidly growing mycobacteria previously has been reported [327,328]. Acid-fast staining of gram-positive bacilli should be routinely included in the identification procedure; if acid-fast staining results are positive, isolates should be sent to a reference laboratory for definitive identification as well as for susceptibility testing.

Case with Error

This case [329] involves a 27-year-old man from India who presented with a 4-month history of fever, anorexia, malaise, weight loss, and erythema nodosum–like lesions on his legs and forearms. A biopsy of an enlarged inguinal lymph node demonstrated caseating granulomata and numerous acid-fast bacilli on Ziehl-Neelsen staining; a portion of this node was sent for mycobacterial culture and molecular analysis. In addition, a skin biopsy of a forearm nodule was done; this revealed acid-fast bacilli that were morphologically typical of *Mycobacterium leprae*. A diagnosis of leprosy was made based on the clinical presentation and the skin biopsy results. However, the lymph node sent for mycobacterial culture and molecular analysis was positive by the Gen-Probe Amplified *Mycobacterium Tuberculosis* Direct (MTD) test (BBL). Although leprosy was still considered to be a correct diagnosis due to the clinical presentation and the skin biopsy findings, the possibility of this patient also having tuberculosis could not be ruled out until the culture results were known. Therefore, the patient was treated for both leprosy and tuberculosis until cultures at 7 weeks as well as additional PCR testing of lymph node material for *M. tuberculosis* were reported to be negative. The patient's response to leprosy therapy was excellent.

Explanation and Consequences

This case illustrates misidentification of a microorganisim due to a false-positive result from a molecular amplification test for tuberculosis. The Gen-Probe MTD test is a rapid molecular test that uses isothermal transcription-mediated amplification and a hybridization protection assay to detect nucleic acid from *M. tuberculosis* complex in clinical specimens including lymph nodes [330]. This false-positive result led to a misdiagnosis of tuberculosis and 7 weeks of unnecessary antituberculous therapy. Fortunately, there were no adverse effects from this therapy.

A root cause analysis was done to investigate this misidentification. *M. leprae* culture material was obtained from the National Hansen's Disease Programs at Louisiana State University; these were tested with the Gen-Probe MTD test and were positive at a concentration of 5×10^5 organisms/mL, but were indeterminate at a concentration of 5×10^4 organisms/mL. The investigators concluded that a high concentration of *M. leprae* in a clinical specimen could lead to a false-positive result with the Gen-Probe MTD test [329].

Conventional diagnosis of mycobacterial infection uses acid-fast staining, culture, and phenotypic characterization of culture isolates; cultures may require weeks or months before results are available. Accordingly, nucleic acid probe- and amplification-based molecular methods have been developed for identification of mycobacterial culture isolates as well as for direct detection of mycobacteria in clinical specimens. These molecular methods have greatly reduced the time to diagnosis of tuberculosis [331]. However, molecular methods have their own set of problems as illustrated by the misidentification of *M. leprae* as *M. tuberculosis* in this case.

Case with Averted Error

This case [332] involves a 60-year-old Turkish man with long-standing leprosy with stable cutaneous lesions on his back and left thigh; this patient presented with progression and alteration of old lesions as well as new lesions on his left arm. Biopsy specimens revealed noncaseating granulomas containing acid-fast bacilli. Although exacerbation of his leprosy was suspected, these biopsy specimens were also tested for *M. tuberculosis*, *M. avium*, and *M. intracellulare* using the COBAS AMPLICOR system [333] for detection of mycobacteria. Test results for *M. intracellulare* were repeatedly positive for four different biopsy specimens. Because the clinical presentation of this patient was consistent with leprosy, the patient was treated for only leprosy. Cultures were negative for *M. intracellulare* after 2 months.

Explanation and Consequences

This case, like the preceding one, illustrates misidentification of a microorganism due to a false-positive result from a different molecular test for tuberculosis. The Roche COBAS AMPLICOR system is a fully automated RNA and DNA amplification and detection system for routine diagnostic PCR [334]. The menu of this system includes selected members of the Mycobacterium family, including *M. tuberculosis, M. avium,* and *M. intracellulare.* The clinical microbiology laboratory was unaware of the clinical presentation and not surprisingly utilized this PCR assay as a rapid method to rule out *M. tuberculosis* and other types of mycobacterium. There were no consequences from this misidentification because the clinicians did not act on the result of this test. Instead, the clinicians relied and acted on their clinical diagnoisis of exacerbation of leprosy.

A root cause analysis was done in order to investigate this misidentification. The laboratory utilized 16S rRNA gene primers in close proximity to the COBAS primers (KY 18 and KY 75) and generated amplicons of approximately 600 base-pairs containing the region amplified by the COBAS AMPLICOR *M. intracellulare* test. These amplicons were then identified by comparative sequence analysis using EMBL and RIDOM databases. The highest scores (greater than or equal to 99.7% identity over a minimum of 450 base-pairs) were for *M. leprae.*

In this case and the preceding one, it is clear that the presence of *M. leprae* in clinical specimens tested by two different molecular assays can result in misidentification for other species of *Mycobacterium.* Clinical microbiologists should be aware of this potential for this type of misidentification of *M. leprae* using commercially available MTB molecular assays.

Case with Error

A 1-month-old previously healthy male infant was admitted to a children's hospital with 1 day of fever. On physical examination, the infant had a temperature of 99.9°F, pulse of 142 bpm, and respiratory rate at 32/minute; the remainder of the physical examination was unremarkable. Laboratory values included a white blood cell count of 11,000/μL with a normal differential. A lumbar puncture demonstrated clear cerebrospinal fluid with a Gram stain revealing mononuclear cells and no microorganisms. The cerebrospinal fluid white blood cell count was 74/μL with 6% neutrophils, 40% lymphocytes, and 50% monocytes; the protein concentration was 44 mg/dL while the glucose concentration was 49 mg/dL. The infant was empirically treated with intravenous ampicillin and gentamicin for possible bacterial meningitis as well as with intravenous acyclovir for possible herpes simplex virus (HSV-1) meningitis pending results of cultures and PCR testing from the cerebrospinal fluid. The following day, cerebrospinal fluid cultures were negative, and the ampicillin and gentamicin were discontinued. The cerebrospinal fluid PCR results were positive for HSV-1. In addition, the cerebrospinal fluid and plasma PCR results were positive for enterovirus. The clinicians felt that enteroviral meningitis was a more likely diagnosis and repeated the lumbar puncture for repeat PCR testing for HSV-1; this PCR test was negative. A repeat PCR assay on the first cerebrospinal fluid was also negative for HSV-1. The positive result for HSV-1 was thus considered to be a false-positive result due to PCR amplification carryover contamination. The acyclovir, which had been continued pending the results of the second lumbar puncture, was discontinued. The child had done well in the hospital and was discharged.

Explanation and Consequences

This case illustrates a well-known problem with PCR testing in the clinical microbiology laboratory, which is PCR amplification carryover contamination and subsequent false-positive results [335,336]. In this case, the false-positive HSV-1 result led to a repeated lumbar puncture as well as an extra day of empiric therapy with intravenous acyclovir. Fortunately, there were no adverse effects from this therapy.

A root cause analysis was done, and no specific, preventable source of the PCR amplification carryover contamination was found. However, the procedure for the PCR assay for HSV-1 was modified to include a repeat assay for any positive results. This will not prevent PCR amplification carryover contamination, but will reduce the likelihood of a false-positive result being reported.

Over the past two decades PCR assays and other DNA/RNA amplification techniques have been utilized in clinical microbiology laboratories. Unfortunately, the exquisite sensitivity of these assays makes them vulnerable to contamination [335,336]. Potential sources of contamination include large numbers of target microorganisms/virions in clinical specimens as well as repeated amplification of the same target sequence leading to accumulation of amplification product in the laboratory environment. The accumulation of amplification product is a critical issue and, if uncontrolled, will lead to contamination of laboratory reagents, equipment, and even the ventilation system [337]. Accordingly, clinical microbiology laboratories utilizing PCR for diagnostic purposes have established protocols to minimize this problem [335–337]. Nevertheless, false-positive results from PCR amplification carryover contamination in molecular assays continues to occasionally occur despite the best efforts of a laboratory. When a false-positive result occurs and is recognized as in this case, a corrected report should be issued. In addition, a root cause analysis should be to done to be sure that there is no recurring systems issue that can be corrected. Finally, communication with clinicians about amplification carryover contamination in a PCR assay is very important; many clinicians do not fully understand this issue and may attribute such false positives to technologist error.

STANDARDS OF CARE

■ Misidentification of microorganisms can occur for a number of technical reasons; microbiologists are familiar with these technical reasons for misidentification, but clinicians may not understand these issues.

■ When misidentification occurs and is recognized, a corrected report must be entered into the health record; moreover, the clinicians involved should be called and told of this error and why such errors occur despite best efforts to prevent them.

■ A root cause analysis should be done for misidentification in order to determine if there are any recurring systems issues that can be corrected.

■ Molecular methods such as PCR can assist in the correct identification of microorganisms, but may require additional time; moreover, PCR methods have their own set of problems with false-positive results due to PCR amplification carryover contamination being the most critical problem [335–337].

■ Because some errors caused by misidentification cannot be avoided due to technical reasons, it is important that microbiologists/pathologist maintain clear communication channels with clinicians in order to quickly explain and resolve such errors when they occur.

SUSCEPTIBILITY TESTING ERROR

> ▶ Susceptibility testing error does not frequently occur in the clinical microbiology laboratory, but such errors can happen. Often there is a technical reason for such errors; automated susceptibility testing systems have been involved in such errors.

Case with Error

A 4-year-old boy was admitted to a children's hospital because of the onset of fever several days after placement of a ventriculostomy catheter for management of medulloblastoma. Cerebrospinal fluid obtained from the ventriculostomy catheter demonstrated 400 white blood cells/µL; a Gram stain of this cerebrospinal fluid revealed gram-negative coccobacilli. Emperic therapy with meropenem and tobramycin was initiated based on the results of this Gram stain. In addition, the ventriculostomy catheter was replaced. The source of the fever was confirmed as sepsis and meningitis when both blood and cerebrospinal fluid cultures grew *Acinetobacter baumannii*. The results of susceptibility testing done by the BD Phoenix Automated Microbiology System [297] showed that the *A. baumannii* isolate was susceptible to both meropenem and tobramycin. The child continued to be febrile despite the fact that the ventriculostomy catheter had been replaced and appropriate antimicrobial therapy was being administered. A repeat cerebrospinal fluid culture obtained from the ventriculostomy catheter was positive for *A. baumannii*; susceptibility testing now showed the isolate to be resistant to meropenem although the isolate continued to be susceptible to tobramycin. However, minimal inhibitory concentrations done by broth microdilution demonstrated tobramycin resistance. The antimicrobial therapy therefore was changed to intravenous colistin; this therapy was selected based on reports of successful treatment of children with postneurosurgical multidrug-resistant *A. baumannii* meningitis using this antimicrobial agent [269]. The cerebrospinal fluid subsequently was sterilized with this therapy. Colistin was given for 4 weeks; the child is now doing well and receiving scheduled chemotherapy.

Explanation and Consequences

This case provides an example of an error caused by susceptibility testing. In this instance, the error was related to an automated system for susceptibility testing. Most clinical microbiology laboratories today rely on automated systems such as the Phoenix Automated Microbiology System for identification and susceptibility testing. Such systems can give inaccurate results for selected antimicrobial agents and microorganism combinations; aminoglycoside resistance and susceptibility testing errors for *A. baumannii* is one of these combinations [338]. It is recommended that confirmation by a manual method be done for this combination. Indeed, such confirmation showed that this *A. baumannii* isolate was resistant to tobramycin.

The *in vivo* development of resistance of this *A. baumannii* isolate to meropenem may be related to an intrinsic class D oxacillinase belonging to the OXA-51-like group of beta-lactamase enzymes [339] or, more likely, to alterations in porin proteins [340]. The oxacillinase intrinsically found in *A. baumannii* is able to hydrolyze carbapenems such as imipenem and meropenem, but only very weakly.

The performance of susceptibility testing in a clinical microbiology laboratory depends on robust methodology, good laboratory practices, and clearly delineated antimicrobial breakpoints. Moreover, routine susceptibility testing must be checked with both internal and external quality control programs. At one time, the results of susceptibility testing were so disconnected from actual clinical outcomes that one microbiologist was compelled to ask "*In vitro* veritas?" [341]. Fortunately, this message was heard and improvements began to occur [342]. Today, susceptibility testing has been greatly improved [343] thanks to organizations like the National Committee for Clinical Laboratory Standards (NCCLS) [6], which has been renamed Clinical Laboratory Standards Institute (CLSI). The published standards/guidelines from NCCLS/CLSI have provided the basis for uniform susceptibility testing procedures in the clinical microbiology laboratory [344]. Although there are still occasional errors as illustrated by this case, these errors should be recognized and quickly corrected.

Case with Averted Error

This case [345] involves a 34-month-old boy who was admitted to a children's hospital with fever, diarrhea, dehydration, and a seizure. The child's past medical history was significant for premature birth at 24 weeks; a ventriculoperitoneal shunt had been placed at 4 months of age for hydrocephalus. The child subsequently had been followed by neurology for recurrent seizures. The child's past surgical history was also significant for Nissen fundoplication and gastrostomy tube placement at 32 months of age. On admission, the child's physical examination was significant for a fever of 102°F and tachycardia. Laboratory studies revealed a white blood cell count of 17,500/μL with 81% polymorphonuclear cells; a lumbar puncture was without pleocytosis. Cerebrospinal fluid and blood were cultured, and the child was treated with empiric meropenem. No growth was observed from the cerebrospinal fluid, but the blood culture grew a gram-negative bacillus that was identified as *Enterobacter cloacae*. Antimicrobial susceptibility testing using a disk diffusion method showed resistance to imipenem and ertapenem, which was an unexpected resistance pattern for *E. cloacae*. The pediatricians caring for this child were not convinced that the susceptibility testing result showing imipenem resistance was correct as such resistance was very unusual in an *Enterbacter* isolate. However, this unexpected carbapenem resistance was quickly confirmed by a modified Hodge test [346]. The isolate was susceptible to levofloxacin and tobramycin; therefore, the child's antimicrobial therapy was changed to levofloxacin and amikacin. The child made an uneventful recovery.

Explanation and Consequences

This case illustrates the uncertainty that clinicians and the clinical microbiology laboratory face when the results of a susceptibility test are not consistent with the established susceptibility patterns for a particular species. The availability and reflex use of the modified Hodge test for confirmation of this isolate's unexpected carbapenem resistance was critical for directing proper antimicrobial therapy for this child. Absence of this confirmatory test might have resulted in a medical error if the screening result that showed imipenem resistance was not considered correct based on the established susceptibility pattern of *Enterbacter* species.

In addition to the modified Hodge test, this *Enterbacter* isolate was evaluated for presence of a KPC-carbapenemase. The isolate was submitted for amplification and detection of KPC using real-time PCR; the bla_{KPC-2} gene was detected using specific primers designed to amplify a 185 base-pair region of this gene. Finally, this 185 base-pair region was sequenced in order to determine the KPC-2 type, and the results of this investigation were published to alert other clinical microbiology laboratories of this potential problem [345].

Gram-negative bacilli producing the KPC carbapenemases may only show reduced susceptibility to carbapenems on laboratory testing. The Centers for Disease Control (CDC) recommends that clinical microbiology laboratories perform a modified Hodge test [346] or use PCR testing to confirm the presence of KPC carbapenemases in isolates with reduced susceptibility to carbapenems. Clinical microbiology laboratories must take an aggressive approach to detecting carbapenemases in order to provide clinicians with clinically relevant susceptibility results.

One of the critical functions of the director of a clinical microbiology laboratory [347] is to select and monitor the susceptibility testing procedures and results so that these provide clinicians with relevant information. As resistance is constantly changing, the director must be aware of newly emerging resistance mechanisms and utilize new molecular technologies to detect such mechanisms.

STANDARDS OF CARE

- Susceptibility testing errors can occur for a number of technical reasons; microbiologists are familiar with these technical reasons for susceptibility testing errors, but clinicians may not understand these issues.

- When a susceptibility testing error occurs and is recognized, a corrected report must be entered into the health record; moreover, the clinicians involved should be called and told of this error.

- A root cause analysis should be done for susceptibility testing errors in order to determine if there are any recurring systems issues that can be corrected.

- Molecular methods such as PCR are being evaluated in place of phenotypic susceptibility testing methods, but are not yet widely used; it should be anticipated that PCR methods also would have their own set of problems.

- Because some errors caused by susceptibility testing cannot be avoided due to technical reasons, it is important that microbiologists/pathologists maintain clear communication channels with clinicians in order to quickly resolve such errors when they occur.

Postanalytic Errors in the Clinical Microbiology Laboratory

OVERVIEW

The postanalytic phase in laboratory testing includes the reporting of the laboratory result to the clinician as well as the clinician's interpretation of that result. Both facets will be addressed briefly in this overview.

Reporting laboratory results has received a great deal of attention since the early 1970s when the concept of critical values in laboratory medicine was first introduced [348–350]. This concept has been expanded to include a vital value [313]. A *vital value* is defined as a laboratory result that is just as important as a critical value, but one for which timing is not as crucial. Many of the test results from the clinical microbiology laboratory logically can be defined as a vital value. Microbiology test results that are of vital value require timely notification of the healthcare provider; most microbiology laboratories call nurses or physicians for such results.

Notification of the healthcare provider for critical values has become an established laboratory policy in all medical centers [349,350]. Indeed, physician communication has become a focal point in efforts to promote patient safety by preventing medical errors [314]. Timely communication of important laboratory data has long been recognized as essential for providing optimal healthcare.

The responsibility for interpretation of laboratory has not been as clear as the reporting of this data. The role of the surgical pathology in the interpretation of histopathologic results has long been recognized [351]. However, similar interpretation of laboratory data by the clinical pathologist has been less clear [352,353], and this concept is only recently coming to the forefront [315,354]. The responsibilities of clinical pathologists, like the surgical pathologist, should extend into the postanalytic phase of the laboratory testing to assist clinicians in reviewing and understanding the results, and often providing an interpretation and/or recommending a future course of action [354,355]. Failure to provide such information may result in a postanalytic error. The examples of postanalytic error that follow are selected from the medical literature as well as from the personal experience of the author and illustrate common postanalytic medical errors from the perspective of the clinical microbiology laboratory.

FAILURE OF CLINICIANS TO CONSIDER AND/OR CORRECTLY INTERPRET MICROBIOLOGY RESULTS

▶ Failure of clinicians to consider and/or to correctly interpret microbiology results is not a frequent cause of medical errors, but does occur. Consultation with infectious diseases clinicians and/or the clinical microbiology laboratory director can help avoid such errors.

Case with Error

This case [356] involves a 30-year-old woman who had lived for many years in New York State and had complaints of chronic abdominal and whole body pain, occasional headaches, and periods of "mental fogginess." She also described a periodic rash that was thought to be a possible "Lyme rash." An infectious diseases physician in New York State who specialized in chronic Lyme disease had evaluated this patient and made a diagnosis of chronic Lyme disease. This diagnosis was based on one PCR assay of blood for the *ospA* gene of *Borrelia burgdorferi*. However, evidence against the diagnosis of Lyme disease included six screening enzyme immunoassay antibody tests for *B. burgdorferi* that were negative, seven Western blot assays that were negative or indeterminate for *B. burgdorferi*, four negative *B. burgdorferi* PCR assays of blood, five negative *B. burgdorferi* PCR assays of urine, and one negative *B. burgdorferi* PCR assay of cerebrospinal fluid. Moreover, a magnetic resonance imaging study of the brain and a lumbar puncture with examination of cerebrospinal fluid had been unremarkable. Despite the predominance of evidence against Lyme disease, this patient received antimicrobial therapy including prolonged intravenous antimicrobial therapy that required placement of an indwelling Groshong central venous catheter. This therapy was discontinued when thrombocytopenia and abnormal liver function studies were noted. Consultation with a second infectious diseases physician was done; this physician thought that this patient did not have Lyme disease. The patient then suffered a grand mal seizure and was admitted to a referral medical center for further evaluation. One day following admission, the patient became confused, fell, and severed her Groshong catheter. She rapidly became unresponsive; electromechanical dissociation was diagnosed, and she died despite aggressive attempts at resuscitation. Following her death, blood cultures drawn at admission were positive for *Candida parapsilosis*. Postmortem examination demonstrated a large *Candida*-infected thrombus located at the tip of her Groshong catheter; this thrombus had caused acute fatal obstruction of the tricuspid valve orifice. At autopsy, there were no findings suggestive of chronic Lyme disease.

Explanation and Consequences

This patient died from a complication of her chronic indwelling central venous catheter, which had been placed for prolonged intravenous antimicrobial therapy for chronic Lyme disease. The diagnosis of chronic Lyme disease, however, was not fully documented [356]. The chronic symptoms of this patient were nonspecific, and the results of her diagnostic evaluation for Lyme disease did not support this diagnosis [356–358]. In this case, the diagnosis of Lyme disease was based on the result of one positive PCR assay out of a total of 11 PCR assays done on this patient; this finding may have been the result of PCR amplification carryover contamination [335–337]. Another similar case with false-positive results for PCR testing for Lyme disease has been reported in the medical literature [359].

The diagnosis of Lyme disease can be difficult [93,96–99, 358,360]; overdiagnosis and overtreatment of Lyme disease is a recognized problem [357,361]. Sequential testing with enzyme immunoassay antibody assay for *B. burgdorferi* and confirmation by Western blot is the most accurate method for ruling in or out the possibility of Lyme disease. This was actually done in the case above, but the results apparently were misinterpreted or ignored by the infectious diseases physician treating this patient.

Case with Error

This case [362] involves a 66-year-old man who was admitted to the hospital because of recurrent fever, arthralgias, and exanthema. The patient had been well until 7 years earlier when a diagnosis of polymyalgia rheumatica was made; treatment with prednisone and methotrexate followed. Two years prior to admission, intermittent episodes of fever with leukocytosis and elevated C-reactive protein had been documented. On admission, the patient complained of weight loss, irregular bowel movements with constipation alternating with diarrhea, polyarthralgias, stiffness of the proximal limbs, episodes of pleuritic pain, and a patchy rash. Laboratory studies included hemoglobin of 11.8 g/dL, a white blood cell count of 22,800/µL with 97% polymorphonuclear cells, an erythrocyte sedimentation rate of 82 mm/hour, and a C-reactive protein of 76 mg/dL. The patient's symptoms of weight loss, arthropathies, and diarrhea prompted an evaluation for Whipple's disease [116,117]. PCR testing from a knee joint fluid specimen and from a duodenal biopsy were positive for *Tropheryma whipplei*. However, a confirmation PCR test using a different technique as well as a 16S rRNA PCR test on the same specimens were negative for *T. whipplei*; moreover, histological examination of the duodenal biopsies did not reveal PAS-positive macrophages. Accordingly, Whipple's disease was excluded, and the patient was assumed to have a systemic inflammatory disorder of unknown origin. During the following 3 months, the patient was treated with indomethacin and prednisone; his clinical status worsened and he eventually died of multiorgan failure. Postmortem examination revealed foamy macrophages in the lamina propria of the small and large intestines as well as in the myocardium, skeletal muscles, bone marrow, and retroperitoneal soft tissue; these macrophages were filled with diastase-resistant PAS-positive particles. Reevaluation of the antemortem duodenal biopsies showed a small number of PAS-positive macrophages. These autopsy findings established a diagnosis of Whipple's disease.

Explanation and Consequences

This case illustrates the difficulty that can be experienced when attempting to make a diagnosis of Whipple's disease [121–123]. In this case, there were contradictory results between PAS staining of the duodenal biopsies and the PCR techniques. The well-known problem of false-positive PCR results for Whipple's disease [121] was also a factor. The authors of this case report conclude that contradictory results warrant antimicrobial therapy with oral sulfamethoxazole/trimethoprim or oral tetracycline as this therapy can result in rapid improvement of the clinical status [362]. In addition, the authors suggest critically reviewing the diagnostic results including meticulous reevaluation of all specimens as well as repeated sampling.

Case with Error

This case [363] involves a 28-year-old male prison inmate with AIDS who initially was admitted to the hospital with headache, fever, chills, and a nonproductive cough. His CD4 lymphocyte count at that time was 24 cells/μL. Physical examination revealed a pustular, indurated nodular skin rash on the torso and extremities [363,364]. A lumbar puncture done on admission revealed a cerebrospinal fluid cell count of 25 cells/μL, a slightly elevated cerebrospinal fluid protein level, and a slightly low cerebrospinal fluid glucose level. Cultures of the cerebrospinal fluid for bacteria, mycobacteria, and fungi were sterile. A biopsy of the nodular rash revealed dermal and subcutaneous microabscesses; a Gram stain of this material demonstrated gram-positive filamentous bacilli. Fluorochrome and Ziehl-Neelsen stains of the nodular biopsy were negative. Based on this information, the patient was treated empirically with sulfamethoxazole/trimethoprim and tetracycline for possible disseminated nocardiosis or nontuberculous mycobacterial infection. The patient's clinical condition improved, and he was discharged back to prison with continuation of his oral sulfamethoxazole/trimethoprim therapy. Shortly thereafter, cultures of the skin biopsy as well as a bone marrow aspirate were positive for *Mycobacterium fortuitum*. Susceptibility testing demonstrated that this isolate was susceptible to amikacin and doxycycline, but resistant to sulfamethoxazole/trimethoprim. The patient was readmitted to the hospital 2 months later; at this time the patient complained of headache, nausea, vomiting, and a stiff neck. The lumbar puncture now revealed a cerebrospinal fluid cell count of 240 cells/µL with 88% polymorphonuclear cells. Antimicrobial therapy with intravenous penicillin and ceftriaxone resulted in no clinical improvement. A third lumbar puncture done 10 days after this second admission because of lack of clinical improvement on intravenous penicillin and ceftriaxone revealed a cerebrospinal fluid cell count of 2,400 cells/µL with 97% polymorphonuclear cells. The antimicrobial therapy was changed to isoniazid, rifampin, ethambutol, and pyrazinamide for possible tuberculous meningitis; his clinical condition improved and he was discharged back to prison. All cerebrospinal stains, antigen tests, and cultures from this second admission were negative. Unfortunately, the fact that skin biopsy and bone marrow aspirate cultures from the first admission had grown *M. fortuitum* was missed. Two weeks later, he was readmitted for the third time with obtundation and nucal rigidity; a lumbar puncture now revealed a cerebrospinal fluid cell count of 1,260 cells/µL with 100% polymorphonuclear cells. It was now recognized that previous cultures of the skin biopsy and bone marrow aspirate had grown *M. fortuitum*. Amikacin and doxycycline were administered, but the patient died 3 days later. Autopsy findings included basilar meningitis; a tissue AFB stain of the meninges revealed branching acid-fast bacilli. Cultures grew *M. fortuitum*. A review of the AFB stains from the skin biopsies done on the first admission also revealed branching acid-fast bacilli [364].

Explanation and Consequences

This case illustrates a number of important points concerning the postanalytic phase of laboratory testing. The first and most obvious point is a careful review of previous culture results; the culture results in this case documented disseminated infection by *M. fortuitum* and also provided the susceptibility pattern for this particular isolate. Clearly, this review of previous culture results was not done, and the opportunity for appropriate antimicrobial therapy was missed. It can be argued that the growth of *M. fortuitum* from the bone marrow aspirate represented a vital value [313] or a sentinel result [7], and telephone notification of this result to the clinicians caring for this patient is indicated.

M. fortuitum infection in immunocompromised patients such as those with AIDS often involves dissemination with multiple skin lesions [364-366]. In contrast, *M. fortuitum* infection rarely involves the central nervous system (CNS) although a similar CNS infection in an AIDS patient has been previously reported [367]. The diagnosis of *M. fortuitum* infection can be difficult as this microorganism stains poorly with fluorochrome stains; therefore, it may not be recognized in smears. Moreover, *M. fortuitum* stains as a gram-positive bacillus on Gram stains and may be confused with diphtheroids or *Nocardia* species. In this case, the initial Gram stain of the subcutaneous micro-abscesses showed gram-positive filamentous bacilli and was reported as probable *Nocardia* species; this resulted in treatment with sulfa-methoxazole/trimethoprim. Follow-up of the skin biopsy cultures was not done.

Case with Error

This case [368] involves a 40-year-old woman who was transferred to the neurosurgical department of a referral medical center with the chief complaint of a 4-month history of headache as well as a computed tomography scan of the head that was suggestive of a brain tumor. Her past medical history was significant in that she had been engaged in prostitution in the past. Her physical examination on admission to the referral medical center was unremarkable; there were no neuro-logic deficits. Laboratory values were remarkable only for a serum Venereal Disease Research Laboratory (VDRL) titer of 1:32, with a positive fluorescent treponemal antibody-absorption (FTA-ABS) IgG test. A brain magnetic resonance imaging (MRI) scan showed a mass measuring 1.6 cm with an ill-defined margin. A diffusion-weighted image revealed a high intensity in the central portion of the mass; this strongly suggested that the lesion could be either a tumor or a brain abscess containing a fluid with high-protein concentration. A proton magnetic resonance (MR) spectroscopy was consistent with a tumor with necrosis rather than a brain abscess. Based on this infor-mation, the patient was diagnosed with a brain tumor, and the mass was surgically resected. Temporal craniotomy revealed the mass to be gray, soft, and attached to the dura of the basal temporal lobe. The mass was completely excised; histopathologic examination noted the central portion of the mass to be necrotic with infiltration by eosinophils. The peripheral portion of this mass had become fibrotic and contained numerous lymphocytic and plasma cells. Occlusion of the small arterioles was noted at higher power views of the mass, and a Warthin-Starry stain of this region demonstrated spirochetes. Postoperatively, a cerebrospinal fluid specimen was found to be VDRL and FTA-ABS IgG test positive. The patient was now diagnosed as having a brain gumma; intravenous penicillin G was given. The patient's headache resolved, and the patient was discharged. Six months later, a follow-up lumbar puncture was done, and the cerebrospinal fluid was noted to be VDRL negative.

Explanation and Consequences

In this case, the patient was preoperatively suspected of having a brain tumor base on imaging findings, but was eventually diagnosed with a brain gumma based on brain histopathology and cerebrospinal fluid analysis. However, this patient's past medical history revealed that she had been engaged in prostitution in the past; a serum Venereal Disease Research Laboratory (VDRL) was positive as was a fluorescent treponemal antibody-absorption (FTA-ABS) IgG test. Based on this serologic information and the imaging studies of the brain, neurosyphilis and a brain gumma should have been considered [369–371]. If neurosyphilis had been suspected in this case, the diagnosis could have been made by analysis of the cerebrospinal fluid; this analysis includes a CSF VDRL and FTA-ABS IgG test.

One might ask if a brain gumma in this case could have been diagnosed without the need for brain surgery. The answer to this question can be found in the following case report from the medical literature [372]. In this case, clinicians suspected a brain gumma based upon a magnetic resonance imaging (MRI) study of the brain. A serum VDRL was positive at 1:16, and the FTA-ABS IgG test was also positive. A lumbar puncture was done and revealed a positive VDRL. Therefore, the patient was treated with intravenous penicillin.

Within 1 week, a loss of contrast enhancement was noted in the lesion on a T2-weighted image; 1 month later the abnormal radiographic findings had disappeared. This case report suggests that surgery is not always necessary for the diagnosis and treatment of brain gumma.

This case also illustrates the potential value of infectious diseases [128,129] and/or clinical microbiology [127] consultations by clinical services such as neurosurgery, which are not as familiar with the diagnostic approach for infections such as syphilis. Such a consultation in this case would most likely have avoided the need for brain surgery in this patient.

Case with Averted Error

This case [373] involves a 47-year-old man who was admitted to the hospital because of fever, headache, rash, and vomiting. The patient had been well until approximately 1 week earlier, when he developed severe pleuritic chest pain and a maculopapular rash on his torso as well as his arms and legs, sparing the palms and soles. His temperature was as high as 39.1°C and was accompanied by chills, diaphoresis, and a throbbing frontal headache. He also had a sore throat and swollen cervical lymph nodes as well as a cough productive of thick yellow sputum. Five days prior to admission, he was seen in the emergency department of another hospital where he was evaluated; his laboratory values at that time included a white blood cell count of 4,900 cells/μL. He was diagnosed as having a viral syndrome and sent home on acetaminophen. His symptoms did not improve, and 3 days prior to admission, he was seen at a medical walk-in clinic where he was found to have diffusely red and enlarged tonsils with a sparse white exudate, palpable anterior and posterior cervical lymph nodes as well as inguinal nodes bilaterally, and brown-gray macules on the trunk and face. Laboratory tests were noncontributory; a heterophile antibody was negative as was antibody (IgM and IgG) testing for toxoplasmosis. He was again sent home and told to take ibuprofen alternating with acetaminophen for fever and to return in 3 days, or sooner if the symptoms worsened. He returned as instructed 3 days later; his symptoms persisted and now he complained of increased nausea and vomiting. He also reported photophobia and neck stiffness. A lumbar puncture was done; cerebrospinal fluid analysis revealed 11 white blood cells/μL with 70% lymphocytes, an elevated protein, and a normal glucose. The patient was admitted to the hospital at this time. His past medical history was significant in that he lived with a single male partner who had been diagnosed with HIV infection 4 years ago. For this reason, this patient was tested for HIV infection. His ELISA was weakly positive, but his Western blot testing was negative for both HIV-1 and HIV-2. However, additional testing was done; quantitative testing for HIV-1 nucleic acids was positive at 45.7 million copies of RNA per milliliter of plasma. A diagnosis of acute HIV infection was made.

Explanation and Consequences

This case illustrates the potential difficulty in diagnosing acute HIV infection as this infection is characterized by a negative or weakly positive ELISA test for HIV, a negative or indeterminate Western blot analysis for HIV-1, and high-level viremia detected by nucleic acid testing [374]. This patient was seen in an outpatient setting two times before finally being admitted to the hospital where this diagnosis was made. Fortunately, the physicians caring for this patient after his hospitalization recognized the need for quantitative testing for HIV-1 nucleic acids to make this diagnosis. The fact that the ELISA test for HIV was weakly positive and the Western blot analysis for HIV-1 was negative did not prevent the correct test from being done. A potential error was thus averted.

This patient initially presented with a classic mononucleosis-like triad of fever, sore throat, and lymphadenopathy. The patient was tested for mononucleosis on his visit to the walk-in clinic 3 days before his hospitalization. In addition, he was tested for toxoplasmosis and parvovirus B19 during his walk-in clinic visit, and after admission was tested for EBV and CMV; these pathogens are among the most common causes of a mononucleosis-like syndrome [375]. This patient's illness persisted for more than a week, and he eventually presented with vomiting, neck stiffness, and evidence of meningitis on lumbar puncture. Although the patient's cerebrospinal fluid was not tested for HIV-1, his meningitis was undoubtedly caused by acute infection with HIV-1.

Acute HIV-1 infection is another recognized cause of a mono-nucleosis-like syndrome [373–376] and should be considered in the differential diagnosis for patients presenting with a classic mono-nucleosis-like triad of fever, sore throat, and lymphadenopathy. The diagnosis of acute HIV-1 largely depends on quantitative testing for HIV-1 nucleic acids. Finally, acute HIV-1 infection presenting as a mononucleosis-like syndrome also must be considered in adolescents as up to half of all new HIV-1 infections occur in this age group [377,378].

Case with Averted Error

This case [379] involves a 30-year-old man who presented with a 10-lb weight loss over a 2-month period as well as a 1-week history of a nonproductive cough. This patient had received an autologous stem cell transplantation as rescue treatment for stage IV nodular sclerosing Hodgkin's lymphoma that had proved refractory to multiple chemo-therapeutic regimens. This patient had no complaints of fever, chills, night sweats, or dyspnea and reported a recent skin test that was negative for tuberculosis. On admission, the patient was afebrile; his physical examination revealed only a few anterior cervical lymph nodes and bibasilar rales on chest auscultation. Laboratory values included a white blood cell count of 2,900 cells/µL with 83% polymorphonuclear cells and a platelet count of 21,000/µL. A chest radiograph revealed small nodular opacities bilaterally; a computed tomography of the chest and abdomen demonstrated bilateral diffuse nodular infiltrates of the chest, hilar/mediastinal lymphadenopathy, and hepatospleno-megaly. Empiric antimicrobial therapy with intravenous moxifloxacin and fluconazole was initiated pending results of blood cultures; these included a lysis-centrifugation technique fungal blood culture and were negative. The result of a serum galactomannan assay [190–192] was positive; the patient therefore was suspected to have pulmonary aspergillosis [189]. The antimicrobial therapy was changed to intra-venous voriconazole. However, the infectious diseases consultant was not satisfied with a diagnosis of pulmonary aspergillosis given the fact that the patient was from Tennessee and had hilar/mediastinal lymph-adenopathy and hepatosplenomegaly, which would be more consistent with a diagnosis of histoplasmosis. Therefore, bronchoscopy was done; bronchoalveolar lavage (BAL) fluid revealed small intracellular yeast suggestive of *Histoplasma*. The antimicrobial therapy was changed to intravenous amphotericin B lipid complex for several weeks followed by oral itraconazole. Results of urine and serum *Histoplasma* antigen testing [8] were strongly positive. Moreover, cultures of the BAL fluid ultimately grew *Histoplasma capsulatum*. Follow-up chest radiographs done 9 months later showed complete resolution of the infiltrates; the patient clinically was doing well.

Explanation and Consequences

This case illustrates another potential problem with interpretation of positive results with the galactomannan antigen test for invasive aspergillosis [190–192]. The serum galactomannan antigen test has been shown to be useful for the diagnosis and management of invasive aspergillosis [192], but has several potential problems with false-positive results. The first cause of a false-positive result is concomitant use of certain antibiotics (amoxicillin-clavulanic acid [187] and piperacillin-tazobactam [188]), while the second cause of a false-positive result as illustrated by this case is disseminated histoplasmosis [379,380]. In this case, voriconazole was started when the serum galactomannan antigen test was positive. Although the data concerning the use of voriconazole for the treatment of histoplasmosis are limited, there is a case report of successful treatment of a histoplasmosis brain abscess with voriconazole [381]. The short course of therapy with voriconazole that this patient received is unlikely to have had an adverse effect and might have been beneficial. In any case, the results of the serum galactomannan antigen test were not considered to be definitive as this patient's clinical picture was more consistent with histoplasmosis than with invasive aspergillosis. Therefore, bronchoscopy as well as urine and serum *Histoplasma* antigen testing were done; these allowed the correct diagnosis to be made.

Galactomannan is a heteropolysaccharide found in the cell wall of most *Aspergillus* and *Penicillium* species [190–192]. The galactomannan molecule consists of a nonimmunogenic mannan core with immunoreactive side chains containing galactofuranosyl units. However, galactomannan has also been found in the cell wall of both the mycelial phase [382] and the yeast phase [383] of *Histoplasma capsulatum* as well as in the cell wall of other fungal pathogens such as *Blastomyces dermatitidis* and *Paracoccidioides brasiliensis* [384]. It is therefore not surprising that cross-reactions can occur when any of these galactomannan-based antigen assays are used [379,380,385]. As pointed out by the authors of this case report [379], the empiric therapy considered should cover both fungal infections until the diagnostic picture becomes clear.

Case with Error

This case [386] involves a 29-year-old woman who was admitted to the hospital because of fever and increasing abdominal pain. This patient had long-standing spastic quadriplegia due to cerebral palsy, but had been in her usual state of health until 2 weeks before admission when she developed intermittent fevers. On the day before admission, the patient had complained of left flank pain, left lower quadrant pain, and foul-smelling urine; she had a history of recurrent urinary tract infections as well as a history of nephrolithiasis. The night before admission, her temperature was as high as 39.1°C and she was brought to the emergency room for evaluation. Because of this patient's spastic quadriplegia and rather complex medical history, which included nephrolithiasis and a ureteral stent, she received a very thorough evaluation over a 12-hour period in the emergency room. The major clinical findings of this evaluation was that the spleen was mildly enlarged, and there were prominent periportal, mesenteric, inguinal, and retroperitoneal lymph nodes seen on a computed tomography (CT) of the abdomen. The complete blood count showed a normal white blood cell count with a normal differential without atypical lymphocytes. Her liver function studies were slightly elevated. During this lengthy evaluation, the patient's abdominal pain persisted and required intravenous narcotic analgesia; the patient was admitted to the hospital for continued analgesic therapy and further evaluation. Over the first 5 days in the hospital, the patient's severe abdominal pain persisted; it was greatest in the left upper quadrant, with radiation to the left flank, and was associated with nausea and intermittent vomiting. On the fifth hospital day, testing for cytomegalovirus, hepatitis B and C viruses, and a heterophile antibody were negative. A repeat CT of the abdomen showed persistent mild splenomegaly with peripheral wedge-shaped areas of hypoattenuation that were thought to represent splenic infarcts. The possibility of splenic infarcts [387,388] in this patient suggested acute Epstein-Barr viral (EBV) infection despite the lack of atypical lymphocytes and the negative test for heterophile antibodies. Therefore, testing for antibodies to EBV-specific viral capsid antigen and EBV nuclear antigen proteins was performed; these were returned as positive on the 10th hospital day.

Explanation and Consequences

This case illustrates the difficulty in diagnosing even a relatively common infectious disease such as mononucleosis when the clinical presentation is not what is usually seen. In this case, the lack of atypical lymphocytosis and the presence of abdominal pain from splenic infarcts are not the usual presentation of infectious mononucleosis. Nonetheless, the subacute illness seen in this young woman with fever, splenomegaly, lymphadenopathy, and hepatitis being the most prominent features should have prompted additional testing for infectious mononucleosis several days sooner that it did [386,388]. Such testing should include antibodies to EBV-specific viral capsid antigen and EBV nuclear antigen proteins [375] despite the lack of atypical lymphocytes and negative heterophile-antibody test results seen early in this patient's course. In this case, the slight delay in making this diagnosis did not cause any harm, but was expensive.

Case with Error

This case [389] involves a 41-year-old woman with a nonlactational recurrent breast abscess. This woman was initially seen with a breast abscess; culture of a fine-needle aspiration specimen grew only *Staphylococcus lugdunensis*. Antimicrobial therapy was deferred because this microorganism was thought to be a skin contaminant. However, the breast abscess persisted for over 4 months until the patient had the abscess surgically removed. The excised breast tissue contained a draining cavity 2 cm in diameter. Histopathologic examination demonstrated that this cavity was lined by granulation tissue, which had marked chronic inflammation with lymphocytes, plasma cells, and rare polymorphonuclear cells. Cultures of this excised breast abscess again grew only *S. lugdunensis*; the patient received postoperative intravenous vancomycin for 2 weeks and has done well.

Explanation and Consequences

This case illustrates lack of recognition of *S. lugdunensis* as a pathogen. *S. lugdunensis* is a member of the coagulase-negative staphylococci and, as such, may not be considered a pathogen. However, *S. lugdunensis* has become recognized as an atypically virulent pathogen with a unique clinical profile [391]. *S. lugdunensis* is a skin commensal and a less frequent pathogen compared to *Staphylococcus aureus*, but clinical infections caused by *S. lugdunensis* act more like infections caused by *S. aureus*. For example, one study [392] evaluated the clinical significance of *S. lugdunensis* isolates identified from consecutive specimens processed during 1 year in a large teaching hospital. This study noted that 86% of these *S. lugdunensis* isolates were clinically significant pathogens. Another study [393] of 229 consecutive *S. lugdunensis* isolates found that 55.4% were isolated from skin infections and 17.4% were isolated from blood and vascular infections. Only 15.4% of these isolates were considered to be true contaminants, which is a similar percentage to that found in the first study [392]. Although coagulase-negative staphylococci are rarely found in a breast abscess [394], this study [390] and another published case [395] demonstrate that such infections can occur.

In this case, there were no serious consequences to the patient despite a delay in definitive treatment for this *S. lugdunensis* breast abscess. However, there might have been serious consequences had this *S. lugdunensis* isolate been involved in endocarditis. Although rare, *S. lugdunensis* is now a recognized cause of endocarditis [396] and can cause destructive native valve endocarditis [397,398]. Clearly, a delay in treatment might have had more serious consequences. Because *S. lugdunensis* isolated from blood cultures in children or adults may indicate infectious endocarditis, coagulase-negative staphylococci from blood cultures should be speciated [399–401].

STANDARDS OF CARE

■ Failure of clinicians to consider and/or correctly interpret microbiology results is less likely in an age of electronic information when the medical literature is available on one's telephone; given this fact, this type of error is less forgivable.

■ When clinicians do fail to consider and/or correctly interpret microbiology results, it is likely to be an oversight; attention to detail is important when considering the volume of information generated by a medical evaluation.

■ Newer molecular tests and/or newer antigen tests are perhaps easier to misinterpret, in part, because of their newness; their sensitivity and specificity may still be evolving.

■ Recognition of the pathogenesis and virulence of microorganisms is constantly evolving; do not assume that a microorganism is not a pathogen simply because it was not recognized as such in the past.

■ Consultation (both formal and informal) with either the microbiology laboratory and/or the infectious diseases consultant is readily available and should be utilized when a clinician is unsure of how to interpret microbiology results; email has replaced the "curb-side consultation" and is very convenient.

4 Summary and Thoughts for Future Direction

Medical errors seen in the clinical microbiology laboratory can occur in any of the following phases of testing: preanalytic testing phase, analytic testing phase, and postanalytic testing phase. The medical literature as well as the author's 30+ years of experience indicate that preanalytic errors are the most common types of medical errors seen in the clinical microbiology laboratory. This is not surprising, as errors in the analytic phase of testing have been addressed for a much longer period of time by quality control programs [1, 2, 5, 6]. The less common analytic errors that do occasionally occur are usually technical issues such as Gram-stain variability that are well known to microbiologists, but may not be appreciated by clinicians. The least common errors seen in clinical microbiology are postanalytic errors. This also should come as no great surprise; analyzing the presence of a microbial pathogen from a culture is not particularly difficult; the pathogen is either there or it isn't. Nevertheless, postanalytic errors do occur as illustrated by the cases discussed in chapter 3. Perhaps it is more germane to ask, "What can be done to reduce clinical microbiology errors in the future?" The answer and proactive direction taken at the author's institution to prevent medical errors [314] is the clinical microbiology diagnostic management team (DMT).

The DMT includes the directors of the clinical microbiology laboratories (microbiology, virology, and molecular infectious diseases) as well as the clinical microbiology fellow, the infectious diseases fellow, the pathology residents, and any medical students that are rotating on the clinical microbiology service. The DMT meets daily for clinical microbiology rounds. These rounds include presentation of a clinicopathological case (CPC) presentation by the fellow, resident, or medical student. This case is often an ongoing Vanderbilt case. In addition, bench rounds are made to identify any sentinel results. A sentinel result is akin to what has been termed a "vital value" [313]. These sentinel results are less time sensitive than a "panic value," but patient care is best served by notifying the clinician of these results by telephone. Examples of sentinel results are as follows:

▨ Unusual or unexpected microorganism
▨ Unusual or unexpected site of detection
▨ Unusual of unexpected pathogen phenotype/genotype
▨ Unusual or unexpected antimicrobial susceptibility pattern
▨ Clinical findings suggestive of treatment failure or refractoriness
▨ Clinical findings suggestive of another underlying pathology
▨ Conflicting, confusing, or ambiguous results
▨ Concern for rapid deterioration of patient
▨ Infection control or public health concern
▨ Situations where DMT can orchestrate involvement of ID or other specialty services for improved patient care

The DMT meets later in the day for specific consultations or new sentinel results identified by the microbiology technologists. The DMT works closely with the pediatric and adult infectious diseases services as well as with infection control practitioners. In particular, as antimicrobial treatment issues, follow-up issues, and infection control issues may arise with a specific patient's sentinel result, the infectious diseases services and infection control practitioners are included in the diagnostic management process.

Another function of the DMT involves internal consultation [315] with other pathology services. In anatomic pathology, the detection of infections or infectious agents by use of cytologic and histologic stains is well recognized [402]. The DMT is available for consultation with AP faculty from surgical pathology, cytology, and autopsy for review of any such stains. Examples of such reviews that might be requested include assistance with frozen section diagnosis [288], assistance with assessment of deep mycoses by morphologic methods [292,293], and assistance with cytological diagnosis [402,403]. In particular, assistance by the DMT with the surgical pathology and cytology evaluations of pulmonary infections [404–406] provides valuable input to AP faculty and also provides a learning opportunity for medical students, residents, and the clinical microbiology fellow. The DMT also assists AP faculty with the molecular diagnosis of infections; such molecular methods can be used on tissue blocks where inflammation has been identified on H&E slides [407–409]. Finally, the DMT can provide assistance with autopsies when infection is suspected [410,411].

As mentioned earlier, the DMT is involved monitoring and intervention for significant results. In the clinical microbiology laboratories (microbiology, virology, molecular infectious diseases), the medical technologists routinely inform their supervisor (and often the pathology resident and/or clinical microbiology fellow as well) of any positive results. Some of these results are considered "call values" and, per the Procedure Manual Call Value Policy, are called to a healthcare giver. These "call values" are reported to the supervisor as well. In particular, those results that are considered unusual or significant are brought to the attention of the DMT. In addition, the DMT makes daily microbiology bench rounds to identify and review any interesting positive results as a part of resident/fellow teaching. The results reported as well as any interesting results seen on bench rounds generate a list of patients for whom an electronic health record review is warranted. The electronic health records available at Vanderbilt University Medical Center [316] allow the DMT to review the clinical notes [412] and thus determine if the clinical medical team providing care for the patient understands and appreciates the significance of the microbiology result. As resident training programs by definition involve patient care delivered by physicians-in-training, the oversight provided by an electronic health record review by the DMT for patients with unusual or significant microbiology results serves as a quality improvement measure, can assess resident training effectiveness, and has the potential to improve clinical outcomes [413].

Finally, the DMT is available for preanalytic consultations for clinicians who wish assistance with a diagnostic infectious diseases problem that involves microbiology testing [351–355]. Often when this preanalytic consultation service is used to establish a diagnosis of an infectious disease, the therapy of the patient is turned over to an infectious diseases clinician. This proactive role taken by the DMT provides a value-added service from the clinical microbiology laboratory and greatly assists clinicians with any infectious diseases problems. Most importantly, it should improve patient care by reducing or eliminating many of the medical errors illustrated in this book [314].

References

1. Bartlett RC, Mazens-Sullivan M, Tetreault JZ, Lobel S, Nivard J. Evolving approaches to management of quality in clinical microbiology. *Clin Microbiol Rev*. 1994;7:55–88.

2. Noble MA. Developments in external quality assessment for clinical microbiology laboratories. *Accred Qual Assur*. 2004;9:601–604.

3. Tunkel AR, Hartman BJ, Kaplan SL, et al. Practice guidelines for the management of bacterial meningitis. *Clin Infect Dis*. 2004;391:1267–1284.

4. Branson D. Problems and errors in the clinical microbiology laboratory. *Am J Med Technol*. 1966;32:349–357.

5. Eilers RJ. Total quality control for the medical laboratory. *South Med J*. 1969;62:1362–1365.

6. Bruck E. National Committee for Clinical Laboratory Standards. *Pediatrics*. 1980;65:187–188.

7. Seifert H. The clinical importance of microbiological findings in the diagnosis and management of bloodstream infections. *Clin Infect Dis*. 2009;48(Suppl):S238–S245.

8. Wheat LJ, Kohler RB, Tewari RP. Diagnosis of disseminated histoplasmosis by detection of *Histoplasma capsulatum* antigen in serum and urine specimens. *N Engl J Med*. 1986;314:83–88.

9. Odio CM, Navarrete M, Carrillo JM, Mora L, Carranza A. Disseminated histoplasmosis in infants. *Pediatr Infect Dis J*. 1999;18:1065–1068.

10. Herzog A. Dangerous errors in the diagnosis and treatment of bony tuberculosis. *Ditsch Arziebl Int*. 2009;106:573–577.

11. Horsburgh CR Jr. Disseminated infection with *Mycobacterium avium-intracellulare*. *Medicine*. 1985;64:36–48.

12. Marchevsky AM, Damsker B, Green S, Tepper S. The clinicopathological spectrum of non-tuberculous mycobacterial osteoarticular infections. *J Bone Joint Surg*. 1985;67(6):925–929.

13. Bjorksten B, Boquist L. Histopathological aspects of chronic recurrent multifocal osteomyelitis. *J Bone Joint Surg Br*. 1980;62:376–380.

14. Christensen JB, Koeppe J. *Mycobacterium avium* complex cervical lymphadenitis in an immunocompetent adult. *Clin Vaccine Immunol.* 2010;17:1488–1490.

15. Schwetschenau E, Kelly DL. The adult neck mass. *Am Fam Physician.* 2002;66:831–838.

16. Zeharia A, Eidlitz-Markus T, Haimi-Cohen Y, Samra Z, Kaufman L, Amir J. Management of nontuberculous mycobacteria-induced cervical lymphadenitis with observation alone. *Pediatr Infect Dis J.* 2008;27:920–922.

17. Habermann TM, Steensma DP. Lymphadenopathy. *Mayo Clin Proc.* 2000;75:723–732.

18. Bazemore AW, Smucker DR. Lymphadenopathy and malignancy. *Am Fam Physician.* 2002;66:2103–2110.

19. Cochran AJ. Melanoma metastases through the lymphatic system. *Surg Clin North Am.* 2000;80:1683–1693.

20. Brown JR, Skarin AT. Clinical mimics of lymphoma. *Oncologist.* 2004;9:406–416.

21. Grossman M, Shiramizu B. Evaluation of lymphadenopathy in children. *Curr Opin Pediatr.* 1994;1:68–76.

22. Scott M. Infections involving lymph nodes. In: Collins RD, Swerdlow SH, eds. *Pediatric Hematopathology.* Philadelphia, PA: Churchill Livingstone: 2001:289.

23. Vassilakopoulos TP, Pangalis GA. Application of a prediction rule to select which patients presenting with lymphadenopathy should undergo a lymph node biopsy. *Medicine (Baltimore).* 1996;79:338–347.

24. Chua CL. The value of cervical lymph node biopsy—a surgical audit. *Aust NZ J Surg.* 1986;56:335–339.

25. Correa AG, Starke JR. Nontuberculous mycobacterial disease in children. *Seminar Respir Infect.* 1996;11:262–271.

26. Alleva M, Guida RA, Romo T III, Kimmelman CP. Mycobacterial cervical lymphadenitis: a persistent diagnostic problem. *Laryngoscope.* 1988;98:855–857.

27. Hansmann Y, DeMartino S, Piemont Y, et al. Diagnosis of cat scratch disease with detection of *Bartonella henselae* by PCR: a study of patients with lymph node enlargement. *J Clin Microbiol.* 2005;43:3800–3806.

28. Rolain JM, Lepidi H, Zanaret M, et al. Lymph node biopsy specimens and diagnosis of cat-scratch disease. *Emerg Infect Dis.* 2006;12:1338–1344.

29. Ginsburg CM. An unusual cause of cervical lymphadenitis. *Laryngoscope.* 1977;87:1180–1181.

30. Meijer JAA, Sjogren EV, Kuijper E, Verbist BM, Visser LG. Necrotizing cervical lymphadenitis due to disseminated *Histoplasma capsulatum* infection. *Eur J Clin Microbiol Infect Dis.* 2005;24:574–576.

31. McCabe RE, Brooks RG, Dorfman RF, Remington JS. Clinical spectrum in 107 cases of toxoplasmic lymphadenopathy. *Rev Infect Dis.* 1987;9:754–774.

32. Yamazaki Y, Kitagawa Y, Hata H, Sakakibara N, Shindoh M, Tmamaki N. Cervical toxoplasmic lymphadenitis can mimic malignant lymphoma on FDG PET. *Clin Nucl Med.* 2008;33:819–820.

33. Gillies MJ, Farrugia M-K, Lakhoo K. An unusual case of a superior mediastinal mass in an infant. *Pediatr Surg Int.* 2008;24:485–486.

34. Grosfeld JL, Skinner MA, Rescorla FJ, West KW, Scherer LR III. Mediastinal tumors in children: experience with 196 cases. *Ann Surg Oncol.* 1994;1:121–127.

35. Simpson J, Campbell PE. Mediastinal masses in childhood: a review from a paediatric pathologist's point of view. *Prog Pediatr Surg.* 1991;27:92–126.

36. Chandor SB, Stemmer EA, Calvin JW, Connolly JE. Mediastinal biopsy for indeterminate *Chest.* lesions. *Thorax.* 1966;21:533–537.

37. Massie RJ, Van Asperen PP, Mellis CM. A review of open biopsy for mediastinal masses. *J Paediatr Child Health.* 1997;33:230–233.

38. Jaggers J, Balsara K. Mediastinal masses in children. *Semin Thorac Cardiovasc Surg.* 2004;16:201–208.

39. Cruz AT, Starke JR. Pediatric tuberculosis. *Pediatr Rev.* 2010;1:13–25.

40. Woods WG, Singher LJ, Krivit W, Nesbit ME Jr. Histoplasmosis simulating lymphoma in children. *J Pediatr Surg.* 1979;14:423–425.

41. Baebler JW, Kleiman MB, Cohen M, et al. Differentiation of lymphoma from histoplasmosis in children with mediastinal masses. *J Pediatr.* 1984;104:706–709.

42. Kirchner SG, Hernanz-Schulman M, Stein SM, Wright PR, Heller RM. Imaging of pediatric mediastinal histoplasmosis. *Radiographics.* 1991;11:365–381.

43. Sehouli J, Stupin JH, Schlieper U, et al. Actinomycotic inflammatory disease and misdiagnosis of ovarian cancer: a case report. *Anticancer Res.* 2006;26:1727–1731.

44. Chatwani A, Amin-Hanjani S. Incidence of actinomycosis associated with intrauterine devices. *J Reprod Med.* 1994;39:585–587.

45. Evans DTP. *Actinomyces israelii* in the female genital tract: a review. *Genitourin Med.* 1993;69:54–59.

46. Spagnuolo PJ, Fransioli M. Intrauterine device-associated actinomycosis simulating pelvic malignancy. *Am J Gastroenterol.* 1981;75:144–147.

47. Fiorino AS. Intrauterine contraceptive device-associated actinomycotic abscess and *Actinomyces* detection on cervical smear. *Obstet Gynecol.* 1996;87:142–149.

48. Atay Y, Altintas A, Tuncer I, Cennet A. Ovarian actinomycosis mimicking malignancy. *Eur J Gynaecol Oncol.* 2005;26:663–664.

49. Akhan SE, Dogan Y, Akhan S, Iyibozkurt AC, Topuz S, Yalcin O. Pelvic actinomycosis mimicking ovarian malignancy: three cases. *Eur J Gynaecol Oncol.* 2008;29:294–297.

50. Samant S, Sandoe J, High A, Makura ZG. Actinomycosis mimicking a tonsillar neoplasm in an elderly diabetic patient. *Br J Oral Maxillofac Surg.* 2009;47:417–418.

51. Somsouk M, Shergill AK, Grenert JP, Harris H, Cello JP, Shah JN. Actinomycosis mimicking a pancreatic head neoplasm diagnosed by EUS-guided FNA. *Gastrointest Endosc.* 2008;68:186–187.

52. Lee SY, Kwon HJ, Cho JH, et al. Actinomycosis of the appendix mimicking appendiceal tumor: a case report. *World J Gastroenterol.* 2010;16:395–397.

53. Cowgill R, Quan SH. Colonic actinomycosis mimicking carcinoma. *Dis Colon Rectum.* 1979;22:45–46.

54. Ergul Z, Hoca O, Karahan MA, Seker D, Hucumenoglu S, Ozakkoyunlu S. A transverse colonic mass secondary to *Actinomyces* infection mimicking cancer. *Turk J Gastroenterol.* 2008;19:200–201.

55. Culafic DM, Lekic NS, Kerkez MD, Mijac DD. Liver actinomycosis mimicking liver tumour. *Vojnosanit Pregl.* 2009;66:924–927.

56. Lang CM, Hofmann WP, Kriener S, et al. Primary actinomycosis of the liver mimicking malignancy. *Z Gastroenterol*. 2009;47: 1062–1064.

57. Dieckman KP, Henke RP, Ovenbeck R. Renal actinomycosis mimicking renal carcinoma. *Eur Urol*. 2001;39:357–359.

58. Simons CM, Stratton CW, Kim AS. Peripheral blood eosinophilia as a clue to the diagnosis of an occult *Coccidioides* infection. *Hum Pathol*. 2011;42:449-453.

59. Harley WB, Blazer MB. Disseminated coccidioidomycosis associated with extreme eosinophilia. *Clin Infect Dis*. 1994;18:627–629.

60. Rolston KV, Rodriguez S, Dholakia N, Whimbey E, Raad I. Pulmonary infections mimicking cancer; a retrospective, three-year review. *Support Care Cancer*. 1997;5:90–93.

61. Nenoff P, Kellermann S, Borte G, et al. Pulmonary nocardiosis with cutaneous involvement mimicking a metastasizing lung carcinoma in a patient with chronic myelogenous leukaemia. *Eur J Dermatol*. 2000;10:47–51.

62. Kathir K, Dennis C. Primary pulmonary botryomycosis: and important differential diagnosis for lung cancer. *Respirology*. 2001;6:347–350.

63. Karakelides H, Aubry MC, Ryu JH. Cytomegalovirus pneumonia mimicking lung cancer in an immunocompetent host. *Mayo Clin Proc*. 2003;78:488–490.

64. Madhusudhan KS, Gamanagatti S, Seith A, Hari S. Pulmonary infections mimicking cancer: report of four cases. *Singapore Med J*. 2007;48:e327–e331.

65. Babayigit A, Olimez D, Sozmen SC, et al. Infection caused by *Nocardia farcinica* mimicking pulmonary metastasis in an adolescent girl. *Pediatr Emerg Care*. 2010;26:203–205.

66. Heller HM, Telford SR III, Branda JA. Case records of the Massachusetts General Hospital. Case 10–2005. A 73-year-old man with weakness and pain in the legs. *N Engl J Med*. 2005;352:1358–1364.

67. Donato AA, Chaudhary A. A 78-year-old man with the "summer flu" and cytopenias. *Clin Infect Dis*. 2009;48:1433, 1479–1480.

68. Prince LK, Shali AA, Martinez LJ, Moran KA. Ehrlichiosis: making the diagnosis in the clinical setting. *South Med J*. 2007;100:825–828.

69. Dumler JS, Madigan JE, Pusteria N, Bakken JS. Ehrlichioses in humans: epidemiology, clinical presentation, diagnosis, and treatment. *Clin Infect Dis.* 2007;45(Suppl):S45–S51.

70. Bell CA, Patel R. A real-time combined polymerase chain reaction assay for the rapid detection and differentiation of *Anaplasma phagocytophilum, Ehrlichia chaffeensis,* and *Ehrlichia ewingii. Diagn Microbiol Infect Dis.* 2005;53:301–306.

71. Martin GS, Christman BW, Standaert SM. Rapidly fatal infection with *Ehrlichia chaffeensis. N Engl J Med.* 1999;341:763–764.

72. Gayle A, Ringdahi E. Tick-borne diseases. *Am Fam Physician.* 2001;64:461–466.

73. Parola P, Raoult D. Ticks and tickborne bacterial diseases: an emerging infectious threat. *Clin Infect Dis.* 2001;32:897–926.

74. Samuels MA, Newell KL. Case records of the Massachusetts General Hospital. Case 32–1997. A 43-year-old woman with rapidly changing pulmonary infiltrates and markedly increased intracranial pressure. *N Engl J Med.* 1997;337:1149–1156.

75. Masters EJ, Olson GS, Weiner SJ, Paddock CD. Rocky Mountain spotted fever: a clinician's dilemma. *Arch Intern Med.* 2003;163:769–774.

76. Dumler JS, Walker DH. Rocky Mountain spotted fever—changing ecology and persisting virulence. *N Engl J Med.* 2005;353:551–553.

77. Eremeea ME, Dasch GA, Silverman DJ. Evaluation of a PCR assay for quantification of *Rickettsia rickettsii* and closely related spotted fever group rickettsiae. *J Clin Microbiol.* 2003;41:5466–5472.

78. Eshoo MW, Crowder CD, Li H, et al. Detection and identification of *Ehrlichia* species in blood by use of PCR and electrospray ionization mass spectrometry. *J Clin Microbiol.* 2010;48:472–478.

79. Kaufmann JM, Zaenglein AL, Kaul A, Chang MW. Fever and rash in a 3-year-old girl: Rocky Mountain spotted fever. *Cutis.* 2002;70:165–168.

80. O'Reilly M, Paddock C, Elchos B, Goddard J, Childs J, Currie M. Physician knowledge of the diagnosis and management of Rocky Mountain spotted fever: Mississippi, 2002. *Ann N Y Acad Sci.* 2003;990:295–301.

81. Cragun WC, Barlett BL, Ellis MW, et al. The expanding spectrum of escar-associated rickettsioses in the United States. *Arch Dermatol.* 2010;146:641–648.

82. Setty S, Khalil Z, Schori P, Azar M, Ferrieri P. Babesiosis. Two atypical cases from Minnesota and a review. *Am J Clin Pathol.* 2003;120:554–559.

83. Homer MJ, Aguilar-Delfin I, Telford SR III, Krause PJ, Persing DH. Babesiosis. *Clin Microbiol Rev.* 2000;13:451–469.

84. Vannier E, Gewurz BE, Krause PJ. Human babesiosis. *Infect Dis Clin N Am.* 2008;22:469–488.

85. Carr JM, Emery S, Stone BF, Tulin L. Babesiosis. Diagnostic pitfalls. *Am J Clin Pathol.* 1991;95:774–777.

86. Fibin MR, Mylonakis EE, Callegari L, Legome E. Babesiosis. *J Emerg Med.* 2001;20:21–24.

87. Kyriacou DN, Spira AM, Talan DA, Mabey DC. Emergency department presentation and misdiagnosis of imported *falciparum* malaria. *Ann Emerg Med.* 1996;27:696–699.

88. Boggild AK, Page AV, Keystone JS, Morris AM, Liles WC. Delay in diagnosis: malaria in a returning traveler. *CMAJ.* 2009;180:1129–1131.

89. Seabolt JP. *Babesia*: challenges for the medical technologist. *Lab Med.* 1982;13:547–551.

90. Brucker DA, Garcia LS, Shimizu RY, Goldstein EJ, Murray PM, Lazar GS. Babesiosis: problems in diagnosis using autoanalyzers. *Am J Clin Pathol.* 1985;83:520–521.

91. Pershing DH, Mathiesen D, Marshall WF, et al. Detection of *Babesia microti* by polymerase chain reaction. *J Clin Microbiol.* 1992;30:2097–2103.

92. Greer DM, Schaefer PW, Plotkin SR, Hasserjian RP, Steere AC. Case 11–2007: a 59-year-old man with neck pain, weakness in the arms, and cranial-nerve palsies. *N Engl J Med.* 2007;356:1561–1570.

93. Recommendations for test performance and interpretation from the Second National Conference on Serologic Diagnosis of Lyme Disease. *MMWR Morb Mortal Wkly Rep.* 1995;44:590–591.

94. Kristoferitsch W. Neurological manifestations of Lyme borreliosis: clinical definition and differential diagnosis. *Scand J Infect Dis Suppl.* 1991;77:64–73.

95. Olivier R, Godfroid E, Heintz R, Bigaignon G, Bollen A. Lyme borreliosis in a patient with severe multiple cranial neuropathy. *Clin Infect Dis.* 1995;20:200.

96. Barbour AG. Laboratory aspects of Lyme borreliosis. _Clin Microbiol Rev._ 1988;1:399–414.

97. Aguero-Rosenfeld ME, Wang G, Schwartz I, Wormser GP. Diagnosis of Lyme borreliosis. _Clin Microbiol Rev._ 2005;18:484–509.

98. Aguero-Rosenfeld ME. Lyme disease: laboratory issues. _Infect Dis Clin N Am._ 2008;22:301–313.

99. Wormser GP. Early Lyme disease. _N Engl J Med._ 2006;354:2794–2801.

100. Lachance DH, O'Neill BP, Macdonald DR, et al. Primary leptomingeal lymphoma: report of 9 cases, diagnosis with immunocytochemical analysis, and review of the literature. _Neurology._ 1991;41:95–100.

101. Kieslich M, Fiedler A, Driever PH, Weis R, Schwabe D, Jacobi G. Lyme borreliosis mimicking central nervous system malignancy: the diagnostic pitfall of cerebrospinal fluid cytology. _Brain Dev._ 2000;22:403–406.

102. Walther EU, Seelos K, Bise K, Mayer M, Straube A. Lyme neuroborreliosis mimicking primary CNS lymphoma. _Eur Neurol._ 2004;5:43–45.

103. Thompson AJ, Brown MM, Ridley A. _Escherichia coli_ meningitis and disseminated strongyloidiasis. _J Neurol Neurosurg Psychiatry._ 1988;51:1596–1597.

104. Smallman LA, Young JA, Shortland-Webb WR, Carey MP, Michael J. _Strongyloides stercoralis_ hyperinfection syndrome with _Escherichia coli_ meningitis: report of two cases. _J Clin Pathol._ 1986;39:366–370.

105. Newberry AM, Williams DN, Stauffer WM, Boulware DR, Hendel-Paterson BR, Walker PF. _Strongyloides_ hyperinfection presenting as acute respiratory failure and gram-negative sepsis. _Chest._ 2005;128:3681–3684.

106. Shorman M, Al-Tawfiq JA. _Strongyloides stercoralis_ hyperinfection presenting as acute respiratory failure and Gram-negative sepsis in a patient with astrocytoma. _Int J Infect Dis._ 2009;13:e288–e291.

107. Igra-Siegman Y, Kapila R, Sen P, Kaminski ZC, Louria DB. Syndrome of hyperinfection with _Strongyloides stercoralis_. _Rev Infect Dis._ 1981;3:397–407.

108. Segarra-Newnham M. Manifestations, diagnosis, and treatment of _Strongyloides stercoralis_ infection. _Ann Phamacother._ 2007;41:1992–2001.

109. Genta RM. Dysregulation of strongyloidiasis: a new hypothesis. *Clin Microbiol Rev.* 1992;5:345–355.

110. Barnes PJ. Anti-inflammatory actions of glucocorticoids: molecular mechanisms. *Clin Sci.* 1998;94:557–572.

111. Hughes R, McGuire G. Delayed diagnosis of disseminated strongyloidiasis. *Intensive Care Med.* 2001;27:310–312.

112. Case records of the Massachusetts General Hospital. Weekly clinicopathological exercises. Case 35–1971. *N Engl J Med.* 1971;285:567–575.

113. Raoult D, Birg M, La Scola B, et al. Cultivation of the bacillus of Whipple's disease. *N Engl J Med.* 2000;342:620–625.

114. Whipple GH. A hitherto undescribed disease characterized anatomically by deposits of fat and fatty acids in the intestinal and mesenteric lymphatic tissues. *Bull Johns Hopkins Hosp.* 1907;18:382–391.

115. Fleming JL, Wiesner RH, Shorter RG. Whipple's disease: clinical, biochemical, and histopathologic features and assessment of treatment in 29 patients. *Mayo Clin Proc.* 1988;63:539–551.

116. Durand DV, Lecomte C, Cathebras P, Rousset H, Godeau P. Whipple disease. Clinical review of 52 cases. *Medicine.* 1997;76:170–184.

117. Fenollar F, Puechal X, Raoult D. Whipple's disease. *N Engl J Med.* 2007;356:55–66.

118. Wolfert AL, Wright JE. Whipple's disease presenting as sarcoidosis and valvular heart disease. *South Med J.* 1999;92:820–825.

119. Dzirto L, Hubner M, Muller C, et al. A mimic of sarcoidosis. *Lancet.* 2007;369:1832.

120. Fenollar F, Fournier PE, Robert C, Raoult D. Use of genome selected repeated sequences increases the sensitivity of PCR detection of *Tropheryma whipplei. J Clin Microbiol.* 2004;42:401–403.

121. Ehrbar HU, Bauerfeind P, Dutly F, Koelz HR, Altwegg M. PCR-positive tests for *Tropheryma whipplei* in patients without Whipple's disease. *Lancet.* 1999;353:2214.

122. Fenollar F, Laouira S, Lepidi H, Rolain J, Raoult D. Value of *Tropheryma whipplei* quantitative polymerase chain reaction assay for the diagnosis of Whipple disease: usefulness of saliva and stool specimens for first-line screening. *Clin Infect Dis.* 2008;47:659–667.

123. Fenoliar F, Ampoux B, Raoult D. A paradoxical *Tropheryma whipplei* Western blot differentiates patients with Whipple disease from asymptomatic carriers. *Clin Infect Dis*. 2009;49:717–723.

124. Doig GS, Simpson F. Efficient literature searching: a core skill for the practice of evidence-base medicine. *Intensive Care Med*. 2003;29:2119–2127.

125. Ebbert JO, Dupras DM, Egwin PJ. Searching the medical literature using PubMed: a tutorial. *Mayo Clin Proc*. 2003;78:87–91.

126. *UpToDate.com*. Accessed October 4, 2010.

127. Thompson RB Jr, Peterson LR. Role of the clinical microbiology laboratory in the diagnosis of infections. *Cancer Treat Res*. 1998;96:143–165.

128. Duncan CJ, Gallacher K, Kennedy DH, Fox R, Seaton RA, MacConnachie AA. Infectious disease telephone consultations: numerous, varied, and an important educational resource. *J Infect*. 2007;54:515–516.

129. Grace C, Alston WK, Ramundo M, Polish L, Kirkpatric B, Huston C. The complexity, relative value, and financial worth of curbside consultations in an academic infectious diseases unit. *Clin Infect Dis.*. 2010;51:651–655.

130. Wadei H, Alangaden GJ, Sillix DH, et al. West Nile virus encephalitis: an emerging disease in renal transplant recipients. *Clin Transplant*. 2004;18:753–758.

131. Centers for Disease Control and Prevention. Final 2009 West Nile virus activity in the United States. Centers for Disease Control and Prevention, Atlanta, Georgia. http://www.cdc.gov/ncidod/dvbid/ westnile/surv&controlCaseCount09_detailed.htm. Accessed October 4, 2010.

132. Tilley PAG, Fox JD, Jayaraman GC, Preiksaitis JK. Nucleic acid testing for West Nile virus RNA in plasma enhances rapid diagnosis of acute infection in symptomatic patients. *J Infect Dis*. 2006;193:1361–1364.

133. Bush MP, Kleinman SH, Tobler LH, et al. Virus and antibody dynamics in acute West Nile virus infection. *J Infect Dis*. 2008;198:984–993.

134. Kapoor H, Signs K, Somsel P, Downes FP, Clark PA, Massey JP. Persistence of West Nile virus (WNV) IgM antibodies in cerebrospinal fluid from patients with CNS disease. *J Clin Virol*. 2004;31:289–291.

135. Prince HE, Calma J, Pham T, Seaton BL. Frequency of missed cases of probable acute West Nile virus (WNV) infection when testing for WNV RNA alone or WNV immunoglobulin M alone. *Clin and Vaccine Immunol.* 2009;16:587–588.

136. Rossi SL, Ross TM, Evans JD. West Nile virus. *Clin Lab Med.* 2010;30:47–65.

137. Sokol DK, Kleiman MB, Garg BP. LaCrosse viral encephalitis mimics herpes simplex viral encephalitis. *Pediatr Neurol.* 2001;25:413–415.

138. Calisher CH. Medically important arboviruses of the United States and Canada. *Clin Microbiol Rev.* 1994;7:89–116.

139. Wurtz R, Paleologos N. LaCrosse encephalitis presenting like herpes simplex encephalitis in an immunocompromised adult. *Clin Infect Dis.* 2000;31:1284–1287.

140. Dykers TI, Brown KL, Gundersen CB, Beaty BJ. Rapid diagnosis of LaCrosse encephalitis: detection of specific immunoglobulin M in cerebrospinal fluid. *J Clin Microbiol.* 1985;22:740–744.

141. Centers for Disease Control and Prevention. Case definitions for infectious conditions under public health surveillance. *MMWR Morb Mortal Wkly Rep.* 1997;46:12–13.

142. Lambert AJ, Nasci RS, Cropp BC, et al. Nucleic acid amplification assays for detection of La Crosse virus RNA. *J Clin Microbiol.* 2005;43:1885–1889.

143. Feder HM, Whitaker DL. Misdiagnosis of erythema migrans. *Am J Med.* 1995;99:412–419.

144. Malane MS, Grant-Keis JM, Feder HM Jr, Lugar SW. Diagnosis of Lyme disease based on dermatologic manifestation. *Ann Intern Med.* 1991;114:490–498.

145. Dandache P, Nadelman RB. Erythema migrans. *Infect Dis Clin N Am.* 2008;22:235–260.

146. Egberts F, Moller M, Proksch E, Schwarz T. Multiple erythema migrans—manifestation of systemic cutaneous borreliosis. *J Dtsch Dermatol Ges.* 2008;6:350–353.

147. Sperber SJ, Schleupner CJ. Leptospirosis: a forgotten cause of aseptic meningitis and multisystem febrile illness. *South Med J.* 1989;10:1285–1288.

148. Feigin RD, Lobes LA, Anderson D, Pickering L. Human leptospirosis from immunized dogs. *Ann Intern Med.* 1973;79:777–785.

149. Lecour H, Miranda M, Margo C, Rocha A, Goncalves V. Human leptospirosis—a review of 50 cases. *Infection.* 1989;17:8–12.

150. Bharti AR, Nally JE, Ricaldi JN, et al. Leptospirosis: a zoonotic disease of global importance. *Lancet Infect Dis.* 2003;3:757–771.

151. Vijayachari P, Sugunan AP, Shriram AN. Leptospirosis: an emerging global public health problem. *J Biosci.* 2008;33:557–569.

152. Easton A. Leptospirosis in Philippine floods. *BMJ.* 1999;319:212.

153. Ricaldi JN, Vinetz JM. Lepatospirosis in the tropics and in travelers. *Curr Infect Dis Rep.* 2006;8:51–58.

154. Lo Re V III, Gluckman SJ. Fever in the returned traveler. *Am J Fam Physician.* 2003;68:1343–1350.

155. Bajani MD, Ashvord DA, Bragg SL, et al. Evaluation of four commercially available rapid serologic test for diagnosis of leptospirosis. *J Clin Microbiol.* 2003;41:802–809.

156. Ahmed A, Engelberts MF, Boer KR, Ahmed N, Harskeer RA. Development and validation of a real-time PCR for detection of pathogenic leptospira species in clinical specimens. *PLoS One.* 2009;4:e7093.

157. Al-Eissa Y, Al-Zamil F, Al-Mugeiren M, Al-Rasheed S, Al-Sanie A, Al-Mazyad A. Childhood brucellosis: a deceptive infectious disease. *Scand J Infect Dis.* 1991;23:129–133.

158. Franco MP, Mulder M, Gilman RH, Smits HL. Human brucellosis. *Lancet Infect Dis.* 2007;7:775–786.

159. Araj GF. Human brucellosis: a classical infectious disease with persistent diagnostic challenges. *Clin Lab Sci.* 1999;12:207–212.

160. Araj GF. Update on laboratory diagnosis of human brucellosis. *Int J Antimicrob Agents.* 2010;36(Suppl 1):S12–S17.

161. Al Dalhouk S, Tomaso H, Nockler K, Neubauer H, Frangoulidis D. Laboratory-based diagnosis of brucellosis—a review of the literature. Part I: techniques for direct detection and identification of *Brucella* spp. *Clin Lab.* 2003;49:487–505.

162. Robichaud S, Libman M, Behr M, Rubin E. Prevention of laboratory-acquired brucellosis. *Clin Infect Dis.* 2004;38:e119–e122.

163. Ozturk R, Mert A, Kocak F, et al. The diagnosis of brucellosis by use of BACTEC 9240 blood culture system. *Diagn Microbiol Infect Dis.* 2002;44:133–135.

164. Mantur BG, Malimani MS, Bidari LH, Akki AS, Tikare NV. Bacteremia is as unpredictable as clinical manifestations in human brucellosis. *Int J Infect Dis.* 2008;12:303–307.

165. Al Dalhouk S, Tomaso H, Nockler K, Neubauer H, Frangoulidis D. Laboratory-based diagnosis of brucellosis—a review of the literature. Part II: serological tests for brucellosis. *Clin Lab.* 2003;49:577–589.

166. Wernaers P, Handelberg F. Brucellar arthritis of the knee: a case report with delayed diagnosis. Acta Orthop Belg. 2007;73:795–798.

167. Centers for Disease Control and Prevention. *Brucella suis* infections associated with feral swine hunting—three states, 2007–2008. *MMWR Morb Mortal Wkly Rep.* 2009;58:618–621.

168. Uyeki TM, Sharma A, Branda JA. Case records of the Massachusetts General Hospital. Case 40–2009. A 29-year-old man with fever and respiratory failure. *N Engl J Med.* 2009;36:2558–2569.

169. Dexler JF, Helmer A, Kirberg H, et al. Poor clinical sensitivity of rapid antigen testing for influenza A pandemic (H1N1) 2009 virus. *Emerg Infect Dis.* 2009;15:1662–1664.

170. Uyeki TM, Prasad R, Bukotich C, et al. Low sensitivity of rapid diagnostic tests for influenza. *Clin Infect Dis.* 2009;48:e89–e92.

171. Harper SA, Bradley JS, Englund JA, et al. Seasonal influenza in adults and children—diagnosis, treatment, chemoprophylaxis, and institutional outbreak management: clinical practice guidelines of the Infectious Diseases Society of America. *Clin Infect Dis.* 2009;48:1003–1032.

172. Centers for Disease Control and Prevention. *Updated Interim Recommendations for the Clinical Use of Antiviral Medications in the Treatment and Prevention of Influenza for the 2009–2010 Season.* Atlanta, GA: Centers for Disease Control and Prevention; 2009.

173. To KK, Cheng VC, Tang BS, Fan YW, Yuen KY. False-negative cerebrospinal fluid cryptococcal antigen test due to small-colony variants of *Cyrptococcus neoformans* meningitis in a patient with cystopleural shunt. *Scand J Infect Dis.* 2006;38:1110–1114.

174. Berlin L, Pincus JH. Cryptcoccal meningitis. False-negative antigen test results and cultures in nonimmunosuppressed patients. *Arch Neurol.* 1989;46:1312–1316.

175. Currie BP, Freundlich LF, Soto MA, Casadevall A. False-negative cerebrospinal fluid cryptococcal latex agglutination test for patients with culture-positive cryptococcal meningitis. *J Clin Microbiol.* 1993;31:2519–2522.

176. Saha DC, Xess I, Jain N. Evaluation of conventional & serological methods for rapid diagnosis of cryptococcus. *Indian J Med Res.* 2008;127:483–488.

177. Sugiura Y, Homma M, Yamamoto T. Difficulty in diagnosing chronic meningitis caused by capsule-deficient *Cryptococcus neoformans.* *J Neurol Neurosurg Psychiatry.* 2005;76:1460–1461.

178. Ecevit IZ, Clancy CJ, Schmalfuss IM, Nguyen MH. The poor prognosis of central nervous system cryptococcosis among nonimmunosuppressed patients: a call for better disease recognition and evaluation of adjuncts to antifungal therapy. *Clin Infect Dis.* 2006;42:1443-1447.

179. Heelan JS, Corpus L, Kessimian N. False-positive reaction in the latex agglutination test for *Cryptococcus neoformans* antigen. *J Clin Microbiol.* 1991;29:1260–1261.

180. Widmer A, Hohl P, Dirnhofer S, Brassetti S, Marsch S, Frei R. *Legionella bozemanii*, an elusive agent of fatal cavitary pneumonia. *Infection.* 2007;35:180–181.

181. Murdoch DR. Diagnosis of *Legionella* infection. *Clin Infect Dis.* 2003;36:64–69.

182. Newton HJ, Ang DKY, van Driel IR, Hartland EL. Molecular pathogenesis of infections caused by *Legionella pneumophila.* *Clin Microbiol Rev.* 2010;23:274–298.

183. Muder RR, Yu BL. Infection due to *Legionella* species other than *L. pneumophila. Clin Infect Dis.* 2002;35:990–998.

184. Taylor TH, Albrecht MA. *Legionella bozemanii* cavitary pneumonia poorly responsive to erythromycin: case report and review. *Clin Infect Dis.* 1995;20:329–334.

185. Plouffe JF, File TM, Breiman RF, et al. Reevaluation of the definition of Legionnaires' disease: use of the urinary antigen assay; Community Based Pneumonia Incidence Study Group. *Clin Infect Dis.* 1995;20:1286–1291.

186. DeForges L, Legrand P, Tankovic J, Brun-Buisson C, Lang P, Sousy CJ. Case of false-positive results of the urine antigen test for *Legionella pneumophila. Clin Infect Dis.* 1999;29:953–954.

187. Mattei D, Rapezzi D, Mordini N, et al. False-positive *Aspergillus* galactomannan enzyme-linked immunosorbent assay result *in vivo* during amoxicillin-clavulanic acid treatment. *J Clin Microbiol.* 2004;42:5262–5263.

188. Sulahian A, Touratier S, Ribaud P. False positive test for *Aspergillus* antigenemia related to concomitant administration of piperacillin and tazobactam. *N Engl J Med.* 2003;349:2366–2367.

189. Atge JP. *Aspergillus fumigatus* and aspergillosis. *Clin Microbiol Rev.* 1999;12:310–350.

190. Hope WW, Walsh TJ, Denning DW. Laboratory diagnosis of invasive aspergillosis. *Lancet Infect Dis.* 2005;5:609–622.

191. Reiss E, Obayashi T, Orle K, Yoshida M, Zancope-Oliveira RM. Non-culture based diagnostic tests for mycotic infections. *Med Mycol.* 2000;38(Suppl 1):147–159.

192. Mennink-Kersten MA, Donnelly JP, Verweij PE. Detection of circulating galactomannan for the diagnosis and management of invasive aspergillosis. *Lancet Infect Dis.* 2004;4:349–357.

193. Ostrosky-Zeichner L, Alexander BD, Kett DH, et al. Multicenter clinical evaluation of the $(1->3)$-β-D-glucan assay as an aid to diagnosis of fungal infections in humans. *Clin Infect Dis.* 2005;41:654–659.

194. Mennink-Kersten MA, Warris A, Verweij PE. 1,3-β-D-glucan in patients receiving intravenous amoxicillin-clavulanic acid. *N Engl J Med.* 2006;354:2834–2835.

195. Adam O, Auperin A, Wilquin F, Bourhis JH, Gachot B, Chachaty E. Treatment with piperacillin-tazobactam and false-positive *Aspergillus* galactomannan antigen test results for patients with hematological malignancies. *Clin Infect Dis.* 2004;38:917–920.

196. Korownyk C, Allan GM. Evidence-based approach to abscess management. *Can Fam Physician.* 2007;53:1680–1684.

197. Brown-Elliott BA, Brown JM, Conville PS, Wallace RA Jr. Clinical and laboratory features of the *Nocardia* spp. based on current molecular taxonomy. *Clin Micro Rev.* 2006;19:259–282.

198. Gosselink C, Thomas J, Brahmbhatt S, Patel NK, Vindas J. Nocardiosis causing pedal actinomycetoma: a case report and review of the literature. *J Foot Ankle Surg.* 2008;47:457–462.

199. Dowell SF, Smith T, Leversedge K, Snitzer J. Failure of treatment of pneumonia associated with highly resistant pneumococci in a child. *Clin Infect Dis.* 1999;29:462–463.

200. Theerthakarai R, Al-Halees W, Ismail M, Solis RA, Khan MA. Nonvalue of the initial microbiological studies in the management of nonsevere community-acquired pneumonia. *Chest.* 2001;119:5–7.

201. Ewig S, Schlochtermeier M, Goke N, Niederman MS. Applying sputum as a diagnostic tool in pneumonia. Limited yield, minimal impact on treatment decisions. *Chest.* 2002;121:1486–1492.

202. Bartlett JG. Diagnostic test for etiologic agents of community-acquired pneumonia. *Infect Dis Clin North Am.* 2004;18:809–827.

203. Musher DM, Montoya R, Wanahita A. Diagnostic value of microscopic examination of Gram-stained sputum and sputum cultures in patients with bacteremic pneumococcal pneumonia. *Clin Infect Dis.* 2004;39:165–169.

204. Mandell LA, Wunderlink RG, Anzueto A, et al. Infectious Diseases Society of America/American Thoracic Society consensus guidelines on the management of community-acquired pneumonia in adults. *Clin Infect Dis.* 2007;44(Suppl 2):S27–S72.

205. Werno AM, Murdoch DR. Laboratory diagnosis of invasive pneumococcal disease. *Clin Infect Dis.* 2008;46:926–932.

206. Isaacs D. Problems in determining the etiology of community-acquired childhood pneumonia. *Pediatr Infect Dis J.* 1989;8:143–148.

207. Jadavji T, Law B, Lebel MH, Kennedy WA, Gold R, Wang EE. A practical guide for the diagnosis and treatment of pediatric pneumonia. *CMAJ.* 1997;156(Suppl):S703–S711.

208. British Thoracic Society Standards of Care Committee. BTS guidelines for the management of community-acquired pneumonia in childhood. *Thorax.* 2002;57(Suppl 1):1–24.

209. Lahti E, Peltola V, Waris M, et al. Induced sputum in the diagnosis of childhood community-acquired pneumonia. *Thorax.* 2009;64:252–257.

210. Efrati O, Sadeh-Gornik U, Modan-Moses D, et al. Flexible bronchoscopy and bronchoalveolar lavage in pediatric patients with lung disease. *Pediatr Crit Care Med.* 2009;10:80–84.

211. Johansson N, Kalin M, Tiveljung-Lindell A, Giske CG, Hedlund J. Etiology of community-acquired pneumonia: increased microbiological yield with new diagnostic methods. *Clin Infect Dis.* 2010;50:202–209.

212. Daily JP, Waldron MA. Case 22–2003: a 22-year-old man with chills and fever after a stay in South America. *N Engl J Med.* 2003;349:287–295.

213. Garcia LS, Shimizu RY, Bruckner DA. Blood parasites: problems in diagnosis using automated differential instruments. *Diagn Microbiol Infect Dis.* 1986;4:173–176.

214. Suh KN, Kozarsky PE, Keystone JS. Evaluation of fever in the returned traveler. *Med Clin North Am.* 1999;83:997–1017.

215. O'Brien D, Tobin S, Brown GV, Torresi J. Fever in returned travelers: a review of hospital admissions for a 3-year period. *Clin Infect Dis.* 2001;33:603–609.

216. Ryan ET, Wilson ME, Kain KC. Illness after international travel. *N Engl J Med.* 2002;347:505–516.

217. Bottieau E, Clerinx J, Van den Enden E, et al. Fever after a stay in the tropics: diagnostic predictors of the leading tropical conditions. *Medicine.* 2007;86:18–25.

218. Sandhu G, Ranade A, Ramsinghani P, Noel C. Influenza-like illness as an atypical presentation of *falciparum* malaria in a traveler from Africa. *J Emerg Med.* In press.

219. Kain KC, Harrington MA, Tennyson S, Keystone JS. Imported malaria: prospective analysis of problems in diagnosis and management. *Clin Infect Dis.* 1998;27:142–149.

220. D'Acremont V, Landry P, Mueller I, Pecoud A, Genton B. Clinical and laboratory predictors of imported malaria in an outpatient setting: an aid to medical decision making in returning travelers with fever. *Am J Trop Med Hyg.* 2002;66:481–486.

221. Doherty JF, Grant AD, Brycesson AD. Fever as the presenting complaint of travelers returning from the tropics. *QJM.* 1995;88:277–281.

222. Jaakkola J, Kehl D. Hematogenous calcaneal osteomyelitis in children. *J Pediatr Orthop.* 1999;19:699–704.

223. De Champs C, Le Seaux S, Dubost JJ, Boisgard S, Sauvezle B, Sirot J. Isolation of *Pantoea agglomerans* in two cases of septic monoarthritis after plant thorn and wood sliver injuries. *J Clin Microbiol.* 2000;38:460–461.

224. Lopez Martinez R, Mendez Tovar LJ. Chromoblastomycosis. *Clin Dermatol.* 2007;25:188–194.

225. Son YM, Kang HK, Na SY, et al. Chromoblastomycosis caused by *Phialophora richardsiae*. *Ann Dermatol.* 2010;22:362–366.

226. Pitrak DL, Koneman EW, Estupinan RC, Jackson J. *Phialophora richardsiae* infection in humans. *Rev Infect Dis.* 1988;10:1195–1203.

227. Yangco BG, TeStrake E, Okafor J. *Phialophora richardsiae* isolated from infected human bone: morphological, physiological and antifungal susceptibility studies. *Mycopathologia.* 1984;86:103–111.

228. Sanford CC. Puncture wounds of the foot. *Am Fam Physician.* 1981;24:119–122.

229. Chisholm CD, Schlesser JF. Plantar puncture wounds: controversies and treatment recommendations. *Ann Emerg Med.* 1989;18:1352–1357.

230. Inaba AS, Zukin DD, Perro M. An update on the evaluation and management of plantar puncture wounds and *Pseudomonas* osteomyelitis. *Pediatr Emerg Care.* 1992;8:38–44.

231. Chang HC, Verhoeven W, Chay VM. Rubber foreign bodies in puncture wounds of the foot in patients wearing rubber-soled shoes. *Foot Ankle Int.* 2001;22:409–414.

232. Miller EH, Semian DW. Gram-negative osteomyelitis following puncture wounds of the foot. *J Bone Joint Surg Am.* 1975;57:535–537.

233. Chang MJ, Barton LL. *Mycobacterium fortuitum* osteomyelitis of the calcaneus secondary to a puncture wound. *J Pediatr.* 1974;85:517–519.

234. Sinnott JT IV, Cancio MR, Frankle MA, Spiegel PG. Tuberculous osteomyelitis masked by concomitant staphylococcal infection. *Arch Intern Med.* 1990;150:1865–1867.

235. Carlos FP, Menry MB. Psoas muscle abscess caused by *Mycobacterium tuberulosis* and *Staphylococcus aureus*: case report and review. *Am J Med Sci.* 2001;321:415–417.

236. Lee IK, Liu JW. Osteomyelitis concurrently caused by *Staphylococcus aureus* and *Mycobacterium tuberculosis*. *South Med J.* 2007;100:903–905.

237. Li JY, Lo ST, Ng CS. Molecular detection of *Mycobacterium tuberculosis* in tissues showing granulomatous inflammation without demonstrable acid-fast bacilli. *Diagn Mol Pathol.* 2009;9:67–74.

238. Colmenero JD, Morata P, Ruiz-Mesa JD, et al. Multiplex real-time polymerase chain reaction: a practical approach for rapid diagnosis of tuberculosis and brucellar vertebral osteomyelitis. *Spine.* 2010;35:E1392-E1396.

239. Gerhardt T, Wolff M, Fischer HP, Sauerbruch T, Reichel C. Pitfalls in the diagnosis of intestinal tuberculosis: a case report. *Scand J Gastroenterol.* 2005;40:240–243.

240. Muneef MA, Memish Z, Mohmoud SA, Sadoon SA, Bannatyne R, Khan Y. Tuberculosis in the belly: a review of forty-six cases involving the gastrointestinal tract and peritoneum. *Scand J Gastroenterol.* 2001;36:528–532.

241. Uzunkoy A, Harma M, Harma M. Diagnosis of abdominal tuberculosis: experience from 11 cases and review of the literature. *World J Gastroenterol.* 2004;10:3647–3649.

242. Khan R, Abid S, Jafn W, Abbas Z, Hameed K, Ahmad Z. Diagnostic dilemma of abdominal tuberculosis in non-HIV patients: an ongoing challenge for physicians. *World J Gastroenterol.* 2006;12:6371–6375.

243. Benevento G, Avellini C, Terrosu G, Geraci M, Lodolo I, Sorrentino D. Diagnosis and assessment of Crohn's disease: the present and the future. *Expert Rev Gastroenterol Hepatol.* 2010;4:757–766.

244. Gan HT, Chen YQ, Ouyang Q, Bu H, Yang XY. Differentiation between intestinal tuberculosis and Crohn's disease in endoscopic biopsy specimens by polymerase chain reaction. *Am J Gastroenterol.* 2002;97:1446–1451.

245. Ibrarullah M, Mohan A, Sarkari A, Srinivas M, Mishra A, Sundar TS. Abdominal tuberculosis: diagnosis by laparoscopy and colonoscopy. *Trop Gastroenterol.* 2002;23:150–153.

246. Tacoveanu E, Dimofte G, Bradea C, Lapascu C, Moldovanu R, Vasilescu A. Peritoneal tuberculosis in laparoscopic era. *Acta Chir Belg.* 2009;109:65–70.

247. Lippi G, Banfi G, Buttarello M, et al. Recommendations for detection and management of unsuitable samples in clinical laboratories. *Clin Lab Chem Med.* 2007;45:728–736.

248. Lippi G, Guidi GC, Mattiuzzi C, Plebani M. Pre-analytical variability: the dark side of the moon in laboratory testing. *Clin Chem Lab Med.* 2006;44:358–365.

249. Lippi G, Blanckaert N, Bonini P, et al. Causes, consequences, detection, and prevention of identification errors in laboratory diagnosis. *Clin Chem Lab Med.* 2009;47:143–153.

250. Lippi G, Guidi GC. Risk management in the preanalytic phase of laboratory testing. *Clin Chem Lab Med.* 2007;45:720–727.

251. Signori C, Ceriotti F, Messeri G, et al. Process and risk analysis to reduce errors in clinical laboratories. *Clin Chem Lab Med.* 2007;45:742–748.

252. Amsterdam D, Barenfanger J, Campos J, et al. *Cumitech 41. Detection and Prevention of Clinical Microbiology Laboratory-Associated Errors.* James W. Snyder, coordinating ed. Washington, DC: ASM Press; 2004:1–14.

253. Musher DM, Schell RF. Letter: false-positive Gram stains of cerebrospinal fluid. *Ann Intern Med.* 1973;79:603–604.

254. Sivalingam SK, Saligram P, Natanasabapathy S, Paez A. Covert cryptococcal meningitis in a patient with systemic lupus erythematous. *J Emerg Med.* In press.

255. Dunbar SA, Eason RA, Musher DM, Clarridge JE III. Microscopic examination and broth culture of cerebrospinal fluid in diagnosis of meningitis. *J Clin Microbiol.* 1998;36:1617–1620.

256. Neuman MI, Tolford S, Harper MB. Test characteristics and interpretation of cerebrospinal fluid gram stain in children. *Pediatr Infect Dis J.* 2008;27:309–313.

257. Bottone EJ. *Cryptococcus neoformans*: pitfalls in diagnosis through evaluation of Gram-stained smears of purulent exudates. *J Clin Microbiol.* 1980;12:790–791.

258. Martin WJ. Rapid and reliable techniques for the laboratory detection of bacterial meningitis. *Am J Med.* 1983;75:119–123.

259. Sharp SE, Elder BL. Competency assessment in the clinical microbiology laboratory. *Clin Microbiol Rev.* 2004;17:681–694.

260. Weinstein RA, Bauer FW, Hoffman RD, Tyler PG, Anderson RL, Stamm WE. Factitious meningitis. Diagnostic error due to nonviable bacteria in commercial lumbar puncture trays. *JAMA.* 1975;233:878–879.

261. Ericsson CD, Carmichael M, Pickering LK, Mussett R, Kohl S. Erroneous diagnosis of meningitis due to false-positive Gram stains. *South Med J.* 1978;71:1524–1525.

262. Hoke CH Jr, Batt JM, Mirrett S, Cox RL, Reller LB. False-positive Gram-stained smears. *JAMA.* 1979;241:471–480.

263. Peterson L, Thrupp L, Uchiyama N, Hawkins B, Wolvin B, Greene G. Factitious bacteria meningitis revisited. *J Clin Microbiol.* 1982;16:758–760.

264. Penn RL, Normand R, Klotz SA. Factitious meningitis: a recurring problem. *Infect Control Hosp Epidemiol.* 1988;9:501–503.

265. Southern PM Jr, Colvin DD. Pseudomeningitis again. Association with cytocentrifuge funnel and Gram-stain reagent contamination. *Arch Pathol Lab Med.* 1996;120:456–458.

266. Ozaki T, Nishimura N, Arakawa Y, et al. Community-acquired *Acinetobacter baumannii* meningitis in a previously healthy 14-month-old boy. *J Infect Chemother.* 2009;15:322–324.

267. Peleg AY, Seifert H, Paterson DL. *Acinetobacter baumannii*: emergence of a successful pathogen. *Clin Microbiol Rev.* 2008;21:538–582.

268. Chen MZ, Hsueh PR, Lee LN, Yu CJ, Yang PC, Luh YT. Severe community-acquired pneumonia due to *Acinetobacter baumannii.* *Chest.* 2001;120:1072–1077.

269. Ozdemir H, Tapisiz A, Ciftei E, et al. Successful treatment of three children with post-neurosurgical multidrug-resistant *Acinetobacter baumannii* meningitis. *Infection.* 2010;38:241–244.

270. Beveridge TJ. Mechanism of Gram variability in select bacteria. *J Bacteriol.* 1990;172:1609–1620.

271. Dubouix A, Bonnet E, Alvarez M, et al. *Bacillus cereus* infections in Traumatology-Orthopaedics Department: retrospective investigation and improvement of healthcare practices. *J Infection.* 2005;50:22–30.

272. Bottone EJ. *Bacillus cereus*, a volatile human pathogen. *Clin Microbiol Rev.* 2010;23:382–398.

273. Drobniewski FA. *Bacillus cereus* and related species. *Clin Microbiol Rev.* 1993;6:324–338.

274. Katsuya H, Takata T, Ishikawa T, et al. A patient with acute myeloid leukemia who developed fatal pneumonia caused by carbapenem-resistant *Bacillus cereus. J Infect Chemother.* 2009;15:39–41.

275. Healy DP, Gardner JC, Puthoff BK, Kagan RJ, Neely AN. Antibiotic-mediated bacterial filamentation: a potentially important laboratory phenomenon. *Clin Microbiol Newsletter.* 2007;29:22–24.

276. Spratt BG, Cromie KD. Penicillin-binding proteins of gram-negative bacteria. *Rev Infect Dis.* 1988;10:699–711.

277. Barenfanger J, Graham DR, Kolluri L, et al. Decreased mortality associated with prompt Gram staining of blood cultures. *Am J Clin Pathol.* 2008;130:870–876.

278. Rand KH, Tillan M. Errors in interpretation of Gram stains from positive blood cultures. *Am J Clin Pathol.* 2006;126:686–690.

279. Strand CL. Positive blood cultures: can we always trust the Gram stain? *Am J Clin Pathol.* 2006;126:671–672.

280. Hendricks WM. Sudden appearance of multiple keratoacanthomas three weeks after thermal burn. *Cutis.* 1991;47:410–412.

281. Lopez Martinez L, Mendez Tovar LJ. Chromoblastomycosis. *Clin Dermatol.* 2007;25:188–194.

282. Amarzooqi S, Leber A, Kahwash S. Artifacts and organism mimickers in pathology. Case examples and review of the literature. *Adv Anat Pathol.* 2010;17:277–281.

283. Bain BJ. Russell bodies. *Am J Hematol.* 2009;84:439.

284. Haensch R, Seeliger H. Problems of differential diagnosis of blastomyces and Russell bodies. *Arch Dermatol Res.* 1981;270:381–385.

285. Patterson JW. An extracellular body of plasma cell origin in inflammatory infiltrates within the dermis. *Am J Dermatopathol.* 1986;8:117–123.

286. Ashford RU, Scolyer PA, McCarthy SW, Boner SF, Karim RZ, Stalley PD. The role of intra-operative pathological evaluation in the management of musculoskeletal tumors. *Recent Results Cancer Res.* 2009;179:11–24.

287. Bui MM, Smith P, Agresta SV, Cheong D, Letson GD. Practical issues of intraoperative frozen section diagnosis of bone and soft tissue lesions. *Cancer Control.* 2008;15:7–12.

288. Coffin CM, Spilker K, Zhou H, Lowichik A, Pysher TJ. Frozen section diagnosis in pediatric surgical pathology: a decade's experience in a children's hospital. *Arch Pathol Lab Med.* 2005;129:1619–1625.

289. Weber CL, Bartley D, Al-Thaqafi A, Embil JM. *Blastomyces dermatitidis* osteomyelitis of the tibia. *Am J Orthop.* 2007;36:29–32.

290. Witte DA, Chen I, Brady J, Ramzy I, Truong LD, Ostrowski ML. Cryptococcal osteomyelitis. Report of a case with aspiration biopsy of a humeral lesion with radiologic features of malignancy. *Acto Cytol.* 2000;44:815–818.

291. Caraway NP, Fanning CV, Stewart JM, Tarrand JJ, Weber KL. Coccidioidomycosis osteomyelitis masquerading as a bone tumor. A report of 2 cases. *Acta Cytol.* 2003;47:777–782.

292. Schwartz J. The diagnosis of deep mycoses by morphologic methods. *Hum Pathol.* 1982;13:519–533.

293. Sangoi AR, Rogers WM, Longacre TA, Montoya JG, Baron EJ, Banaei N. Challenges and pitfalls of morphologic identification of fungal infections in histologic and cytologic specimens: a ten-year retrospective review at a single institution. *Am J Clin Pathol.* 2009;13:364–375.

294. Saccente M, Woods GL. Clinical and laboratory update on blastomycosis. *Clin Microbiol Rev.* 2010;23:367–381.

295. Lazcano O, Speights VO Jr, Stickler JG, Bibao JE, Becker J, Diaz J. Combined histochemical stains in the differential diagnosis of *Cryptococcus neoformans. Mod Pathol.* 1993;6:80–84.

296. Weissert C, Dollenmaier G, Rafeiner P, Riehm J, Schultze D. *Burkholderia pseudomallei* misidentified by automated system. *Emerg Infect Dis.* 2009;15:1799–1801.

297. Stefaniuk E, Baraniak A, Gniadkowski M, Hryniewicz W. Evaluation of the BD Phoenix automated identification and susceptibility testing system in clinical microbiology practice. *Eur J Clin Microbiol Infect Dis.* 2003;22:479–485.

298. Brisse S, Stefani S, Verhoef J, Van Belkum A, Vandamme P, Goessens W. Comparison evaluation of the BD Phoenix and VITEK 2 automated instruments for identification of isolated of the *Burkholderia cepacia* complex. *J Clin Microbiol.* 2002;40:1743–1748.

299. Wiersinga WJ, van der Poll T, White NJ, Day NP, Peacock SJ. Melioidosis insights into the pathogenicity of *Burkholderia pseudomallei. Nat Rev Microbiol.* 2006;4:272–282.

300. Cheng AC, Currie BJ. Melioidosis: epidemiology, pathophysiology, and management. *Clin Microbiol Rev.* 2005;18:383–416.

301. Peacock SJ, Schweizer HP, Dance DA, et al. Management of accidental laboratory exposure to *Burkhoderia pseudomallei* and *B. mallei. Emerg Infect Dis.* 2008;14:e2.

302. Amornchai P, Chierakul W, Wuthieckanum V, et al. Accuracy of *Burkholderia pseudomallei* identification using the API 20NE system and a latex agglutination test. *J Clin Microbiol.* 2007;45:3774–3776.

303. Brigante G, Luzzaro F, Bettaccini A, et al. Use of the Phoenix Automated System for identification of *Streptococcus* and *Enterococcus* spp. *J Clin Microbiol.* 2006;44:3263–3267.

304. Shah M, Centor RM, Jennings M. Severe acute pharyngitis caused by group C streptococcus. *J Gen Intern Med.* 2007;22:272–274.

305. Bradley SF, Gordon JJ, Baumgartner DD, Marasco WA, Kauffman CA. Group C streptococcal bacteremia: analysis of 88 cases. *Rev Infect Dis.* 1991;13:270–280.

306. Brogan O, Malone J, Fox C, Whyte AS. Lancefield grouping and smell of caramel for presumptive identification and assessment of pathogenicity in the *Streptococcus milleri* group. *J Clin Pathol.* 1997;50:332–335.

307. Chew TA, Smith JM. Detection of diacetyl (caramel odor) in presumptive identification of the "*Streptococcus milleri*" group. *J Clin Microbiol.* 1992;30:3028–3029.

308. Whiley RA, Hall LM, Hardie JM, Beighton D. A study of small-colony, beta-haemolytic, Lancefield group C streptococci within the *anginosus* group: description of *Streptococcus constellatus* subsp. pharyngitis subsp. nov., associated with the human throat and pharyngitis. *Int J Syst Bacteriol.* 1999;49 (Pt 4):1433–1439.

309. Vance DW. Group C streptococci: "*Streptococcus equisimilis*" of *Streptococcus anginosus*? *Clin Infect Dis.* 1992;14:616.

310. Bucher C, von Graevenitz A. Differentiation in throat cultures of group C and G streptococci and *Streptococcus milleri* with identical antigens. *Eur J Clin Microbiol.* 1984;3:44–45.

311. Bert F, Bariou-Lancelin M, Lambert-Zechovsky N. Clinical significance of bacteremia involving the "*Streptococcus milleri*" group: 51 cases and review. *Clin Infect Dis.* 1998;27:385–387.

312. Belko J, Goldmann DA, Macone A, Zaidi AKM. Clinically significant infections with organisms of the *Streptococcus milleri* group. *Pediatr Infect Dis.* 2002;21:715–726.

313. Lundberg GD. Is it time to extend the laboratory critical (panic) value system to include vital values? *MedGenMed.* 2007;9:20.

314. Leape LL, Woods DD, Hatlie MJ, Kizer KW, Schroeder SA, Lundberg GD. Promoting patient safety by preventing medical error. *JAMA.* 1998;280:1444–1447.

315. Kratz A, Laposata M. Enhanced clinical consulting—moving toward the core competencies of laboratory professionals. *Clin Chim Acta.* 2002;319:117–125.

316. Stead WW. Electronic health records. *Stud Health Technol Inform.* 2010;153:119–143.

317. Weesner CL, Cisek JE. Lemierre syndrome: the forgotten disease. *Ann Emerg Med.* 1993;22:256–258.

318. Hagelskjaer Kristensen L, Prag J. Human necrobacillosis, with emphasis on Lemierre's syndrome. *Clin Infect Dis.* 2000;31:524–532.

319. Chirinos JA, Lichstein DM, Garcia J, Tamariz LJ. The evolution of Lemierre syndrome: report of 2 cases and review of the literature. *Medicine (Baltimore).* 2002;81:458–465.

320. Centor RM. Expand the pharyngitis paradigm for adolescents and young adults. *Ann Intern Med.* 2009;151:812–815.

321. Han JK, Kerschner JE. *Streptococcus milleri:* an organism for head and neck infections and abscess. *Arch Otolaryngol Head Neck Surg.* 2001;127:650–654.

322. Williamson JC, Miano TA, Morgan MR, Palavecino EL. Fatal *Mycobacterium abscessus* endocarditis misidentified as *Corynebacterium* spp. *Scand J Infect Dis.* 2010;42:222–224.

323. De Groote MA, Huitt G. Infections due to rapidly growing mycobacteria. *Clin Infect Dis.* 2006;41:1756–1763.

324. Repath F, Seabury JH, Sanders CV, Domer J. Prosthetic valve endocarditis due to *Mycobacterium chelonei. South Med J.* 1976;69:1244–1246.

325. Tsai WC, Hsieh HC, Su HM, et al. *Mycobacterium abscessus* endocarditis: a case report and literature review. *Kaohsiung J Med Sci.* 2008;24:481–486.

326. Von Graevenitz A, Punter-Streit V. Failure to recognize rapidly growing mycobacteria in a proficiency testing sample without specific request: a wider diagnostic problem? *Eur J Epidemiol.* 1998;14:519–520.

327. Larkin JA, Shashy RG, Gonzalez CA. Difficulty in differentiating a rapidly growing *Mycobacterium* species from diphtheroids in an immunocompromised patient. *Clin Microbiol Newsl.* 1997;19:108–111.

328. Garg P, Athmanathan S, Rao GM. *Mycobacterium chelonae* masquerading as *Corynebacterium* in a case of infectious keratitis: a diagnostic dilemma. *Cornea*. 1998;17:230–232.

329. Chedore P, Broukhanski G, Shainhouse Z, Jamieson F. False-positive Amplified *Mycobacterium Tuberculosis* Direct Test results for samples containing *Mycobacterium leprae*. *J Clin Microbiol*. 2006;44:612–613.

330. Kerleguer A, Fabre M, Bernatas JJ, Nicand GP, Herve EV, Koeck JL. Clinical evaluation of the Gen-Probe Amplified *Mycobacterium Tuberculosis* Direct Test for rapid diagnosis of tuberculosis lymphadenitis. *J Clin Microbiol*. 2004;42:5921–5922.

331. Balasingham SV, Davidsen T, Szpinda I, Frye SA, Tenjum T. Molecular diagnostics in tuberculosis: basis and implications for therapy. *Mol Diagn Ther*. 2009;13:137–151.

332. Lefmann M, Moter A, Schweickert B, Gobel UB. Misidentification of *Mycobacterium leprae* as *Mycobacterium intracellulare* by the COBAS AMPLICOR *M. intracellulare* Test. *J Clin Microbiol*. 2005;43:1928–1929.

333. Bodmer T, Gurtner A, Scholkmann M, Matter L. Evaluation of the COBAS AMPLICOR MTB system. *J Clin Microbiol*. 1997;35:1604–1605.

334. DiDomenico N, Link H, Knobel R, et al. COBAS AMPLICOR: fully automated RNA and DNA amplification and detection system for routine diagnostic PCR. *Clin Chem*. 1996;42:1915–1923.

335. Borst A, Box ATA, Fluit AC. False-positive results and contamination in nucleic acid amplification assays: suggestions for a prevent and destroy strategy. *Eur J Clin Microbiol Infect Dis*. 2004;23:289–299.

336. Aslanzadeh J. Preventing PCR amplification carryover contamination in a clinical laboratory. *Ann Clin Lab Sci*. 2004;34:389–396.

337. Persing DH. Polymerase chain reaction: trenches to benches. *J Clin Microbiol*. 1990;29:1281–1285.

338. Akers KS, Chaney C, Barsoumian A, et al. Aminoglycoside resistance and susceptibility testing errors in *Acinetobacter baumannii-calcoaceticus* complex. *J Clin Microbiol*. 2010;48:1132–1138.

339. Poirel L, Nordmann P. Carbapenem resistance in *Acinetobacter baumannii*: mechanisms and epidemiology. *Clin Microbiol Infect*. 2006;12:826–836.

340. Clark RB. Imipenem resistance among *Acinetobacter baumannii*: association with reduced expression of a 33–36 KDa outer membrane protein. *J Antimicrob Chemother.* 1996;38:245–251.

341. Greenwood D. *In vitro* veritas? Antimicrobial susceptibility tests and their clinical relevance. *J Infect Dis.* 1981;144:380–385.

342. Stratton CW. Susceptibility testing today. Myth, reality, and new direction. *Hosp Epidemiol.* 1988;9:264–267.

343. Stratton CW. *In vitro* susceptibility testing versus *in vivo* effectiveness. *Med Clin North Am.* 2006;90:1077–1088.

344. Clinical and Laboratory Standards Institute. Performance standards for antimicrobial susceptibility testing. Twentieth informational supplement. CLSI document M100-S20-U. Wayne, PA: Clinical and Laboratory Standards Institute; 2010.

345. Lo A, Verrall R, Williams J, Stratton C, Della-Latta P, Yang YW. Carbapenem resistance via the bla_{KPC-2} gene in *Enterobacter cloacae* blood culture isolate. *South Med J.* 2010;103:394–395.

346. Lee K, Chong Y, Shin HB, Kim YA, Yong D, Yum JH. Modified Hodge and EDTA-disk synergy tests to screen metallo-beta-lactamase-producing strains of *Pseudomonas* and *Acinetobacter* species. *Clin Microbiol Infect.* 2001;7:88–91.

347. Thomson RB Jr, Wilson ML, Weinstein MP. The clinical microbiology laboratory director in the Unities States hospital setting. *J Clin Microbiol.* 2010;48:3465–3469.

348. Lundberg GD. When to panic over abnormal values. *MLO Med Lab Obs.* 1972;4:47–54.

349. Lundberg GD. Critical (panic) value notification: an established laboratory policy (parameter). *JAMA.* 1990;263:709.

350. Dighe AS, Rao A, Coakley AB, Lewandrowski KB. Analysis of laboratory critical values reporting in a large academic medical center. *Am J Clin Path.* 2006;125:758–764.

351. Hutter RV. The surgical pathologist as a diagnostician and consultant. *Am J Clin Pathol.* 1981;75(Suppl 3):447–452.

352. Robboy SJ. The clinical pathologist: physician, not administrator. *Hum Pathol.* 1982;13:788–789.

353. Benjamin DR. Clinical pathologist. A physician's consultant. *Arch Pathol Lab Med.* 1984;108:782.

354. Anastasi J, Ashwood E, Baron B, et al. The clinical pathologist as consultant. *Am J Clin Pathol.* 2011;135:11–12.

355. Laposata M. Patient-specific narrative interpretation of complex clinical laboratory evaluations: who is competent to provide them? *Clin Chem.* 2004;50:471–472.

356. Patel R, Grogg KL, Edwards WD, Wright AJ, Scwenk NM. Death from inappropriate therapy for Lyme disease. *Clin Infect Dis.* 2000;31:1107–1109.

357. Steere AC, Taylor E, McHugh GL, Logigian EL. The overdiagnosis of Lyme diease. *JAMA.* 1993;269:1812–1816.

358. Tugwell P, Dennis DT, Weinstein A, et al. Laboratory evaluation in the diagnosis of Lyme disease. *Ann Intern Med.* 1997;127:1109–1123.

359. Molloy PJ, Persing DH, Berardi VP. False-positive results of PCR testing for Lyme disease. *Clin Infect Dis.* 2001;33:413–414.

360. Sigal LH. Pitfalls in the diagnosis and management of Lyme disease. *Arthritis Rheum.* 1998;41:195–204.

361. Quireshi MZ, New D, Zulgarni NJ, Nachman S. Overdiagnosis and overtreatment of Lyme disease in children. *Pediatr Infect Dis.* 2002;21:12–14.

362. Muller SA, Vogt P, Altwegg M, Seebach JD. Deadly carousel or difficult interpretation of new diagnostic tools for Whipple's disease: case report and review of the literature. *Infection.* 2005;33:39–42.

363. Smith MB, Boyars MC, Woods GL. Fatal *Mycobacterium fortuitum* meningitis in a patient with AIDS. *Clin Infect Dis.* 1996;23:1327–1328.

364. Smith MB, Schnadig VJ, Boyars MC, Woods GL. Clinical and pathologic features of *Mycobacterium fortuitum* infections. An emerging pathogen in patients with AIDS. *Am J Clin Pathol.* 2001;116:225–232.

365. Wallace RJ, Swenson JM, Silcox VA, Good RC, Tschen JA, Stone MS. Spectrum of disease due to rapidly growing mycobacteria. *Rev Infect Dis.* 1983;5:657–679.

366. Ingram CW, Tanner DC, Durack DT, Kernodle GW Jr, Corey GR. Disseminated infection with rapidly growing mycobacteria. *Clin Infect Dis.* 1993;16:463–471.

367. Jacob CN, Henein SS, Heurich AE, Kamholz S. Nontuberculous mycobacterial infection of the central nervous system in patients with AIDS. *South Med J.* 1993;86:638–640.

368. Lee CW, Lim MJ, Son D, et al. A case of cerebral gumma presenting as brain tumor in a human immunodeficiency virus (HIV)-negative patient. *Yonsei Med J.* 2009;50:284–288.

369. Timmermans M, Carr J. Neurosyphilis in the modern era. *J Neurol Neurosurg Psychiatry.* 2004;75:1727–1730.

370. Brightbill TC, Ihmeidan IH, Post MJD, Berger JR, Katz DA. Neurosyphilis in HIV-positive and HIV-negative patients: neuroimaging findings. *Am J Neuroradiol.* 1995;16:703–711.

371. Fargen KM. Cerebral syphilitic gummata: a case presentation and analysis of 156 reported cases. *Neurosurgery.* 2009;64:568–575.

372. Suarez JI, Mlakar D, Snodgrass SM. Cerebral syphilitic gumma in an HIV-negative patient presenting as prolonged focal motor status epilepticus. *N Engl J Med.* 1996;335:1159–1160.

373. Bell SK, Rosenberg ES. Case records of the Massachusetts General Hospital. Case 11–2009: a 47-year-old man with fever, headache, rash, and vomiting. *N Engl J Med.* 2009;360:1540–1548.

374. Kahn JO, Walker BD. Acute human immunodeficiency virus type 1 infection. *N Engl J Med.* 1998;339:33–39.

375. Hurt C, Tammaro D. Diagnostic evaluation of mononucleosis-like illnesses. *Am J Med.* 2007;120:e1–e8.

376. Rosenberg ES, Callendo AM, Walker BD. Acute HIV infection among patients tested for mononucleosis. *N Engl J Med.* 1990;340:969.

377. Aggarwal M, Rein J. Acute human immunodeficiency virus syndrome in an adolescent. *Pediatrics.* 2003;112:e323.

378. Futterman D, Chabon B, Hoffman ND. HIV and AIDS in adolescents. *Pediatr Clin North Am.* 2000;47:171–188.

379. Jones O, Cleveland KO, Gelfand MS. A case of disseminated histoplasmosis following autologous stem cell transplantation for Hodgkin's lymphoma: an initial misdiagnosis with a false-positive serum galactomannan assay. *Transpl Infect Dis.* 2009;11:281–283.

380. Narreddy S, Chandrasekar PH. False-positive *Aspergillus* galactomannan (GM) assay in histoplasmosis. *J Infect.* 2008;56:80–81.

381. Srinivasan J, Ooi WW. Successful treatment of histoplasmosis brain abscess with voriconazole. *Arch Neurol.* 2008;65:666–667.

382. Reiss E, Mitchell WO, Stone SH, Hasenclever HF. Cellular immune activity of a galactomannan-protein complex from mycelia of *Histoplasma capsulatum*. *Infect Immun*. 1974;10:802–809.

383. Reiss E, Miller SE, Kaplan W, Kaufman L. Antigenic, chemical, and structural properties of cell walls of *Histoplasma capsulatum* yeast-form chemotypes 1 and 2 after serial enzymatic hydrolysis. *Infect Immun*. 1977;16:690–700.

384. Azuma I, Kaanetsuna F, Tanaka Y, Yamamura Y, Carbonell LM. Chemical and immunological properties of galactomannans obtained from *Histoplasma duboisii*, *Histoplasma capsulatum*, *Paracoccidioides brasiliensis*, and *Blastomyces dermatitidis*. *Mycopathol Mycol Appl*. 1974;54:111–125.

385. Durkin M, Witt J, LeMonte A, Wheat B, Connolly P. Antigen assay with the potential to aid in diagnosis of blastomycosis. *J Clin Microbiol*. 2004;42:4873–4875.

386. Hunt DP, Thabet A, Rosenberg ES. Case records of the Massachusetts General Hospital. Case 29–2010: a 29-year-old woman with fever and abdominal pain. *N Engl J Med*. 2010;363:1266–1274.

387. Antopolski M, Hiller N, Salameh S, Goldshtein B, Stalnikowicz R. Splenic infarction: 10 years of experience. *Am J Emerg Med*. 2009;27:262–265.

388. Trevenzoli M, Sattin A, Sgarabotto D, Francavilla E, Cattelan AM. Splenic infarct during infectious mononucleosis. *Scand J Infect Dis*. 2001;33:550–551.

389. Luzuriaga K, Sullivan JL. Infectious mononucleosis. *N Engl J Med*. 2010;362:1993–2000.

390. Asnis DS, St John S, Tickoo R, Arora A. *Staphylococcus lugdunensis* breast abscess: is it real? *Clin Infect Dis*. 2003;36:1348.

391. Frank KL, Del Pozo JL, Patel R. From clinical microbiology to infection pathogenesis: how daring to be different works for *Staphylococcus lugdunensis*. *Clin Microbiol Rev*. 2008;21:111–133.

392. Kleiner E, Monk AB, Archer GL, Forbes BA. Clinical significance of *Staphylococcus lugdunensis* isolated from routine cultures. *Clin Infect Dis*. 2010;51:801–803.

393. Herchline TE, Ayers LW. Occurrence of *Staphylococcus lugdunensis* in consecutive clinical cultures and relationship of isolation to infection. *J Clin Microbiol*. 1991;29:419–421.

394. Surani S, Chandra H, Weinstein RA. Breast abscess: coagulase-negative staphylococcus as a sole pathogen. *Clin Infect Dis.* 1993;17:701–704.

395. Waghorn DJ. *Staphylococcus lugdunensis* as a cause of breast abscess. *Clin Infect Dis.* 1994;19:814–815.

396. Liu PY, Huang YF, Tang CW, et al. *Staphylococcus lugdunensis* infective endocarditis: a literature review and analysis of risk factors. *J Microbiol Immunol Infect.* 2010;43:478–484.

397. Burgert SJ, LaRocco MT, Wilansky S. Destructive native valve endocarditis caused by *Staphylococcus lugdunensis. South Med J.* 1999;92:812–814.

398. Van Hoovels L, De Munter P, Colaert J, Van Wijngaerden E, Peetemans WE, Verhaegen J. Three cases of destructive native valve endocarditis caused by *Staphylococcus lugdunensis. Eur J Clin Microbiol Infect Dis.* 2005;24:149–152.

399. Sotutu V, Carapetis J, Wilkinson J, Davis A, Curtis N. The "surreptitious *Staphylococcus*": *Staphylococcus lugdunensis* endocarditis in a child. *Pediatr Infect Dis J.* 2002;21:984–986.

400. Seenivasan MH, Yu VL. *Staphylococcus lugdunensis* endocarditis—the hidden peril of coagulase-negative staphylococcus in blood cultures. *Eur J Clin Microbiol Infect Dis.* 2003;22:489–491.

401. Takahashi N, Shimada T, Ishibashi Y, et al. The pitfall of coagulase-negative staphylococci: a case of *Staphylococcus lugdunensis* endocarditis. *Int J Cardiol.* 2009;137:e15–e17.

402. Woods GL, Walker DH. Detection of infection or infectious agents by use of cytologic and histologic stains. *Clin Microbiol Rev.* 1996;9:382–404.

403. Powers CN. Diagnosis of infectious diseases: a cytopathologist's perspective. *Clin Microbiol Rev.* 1998;11:341–365.

404. Colby TV, Weiss RL. Current concepts of the surgical pathology of pulmonary infections. *Am J Surg Pathol.* 1987;11(Suppl 1):S25–S37.

405. Trumbull ML, Chesney TM. The cytological diagnosis of pulmonary blastomycosis. *JAMA.* 1981;245:836–838.

406. Wilson ML, Winn W. Laboratory diagnosis of bone, joint, soft-tissue, and skin infections. *Clin Infect Dis.* 2008;46:453–457.

407. Molecular identification of pathogenic fungi. *J Antimicrob Chemother.* 2008;61(Suppl 1):S7–S12.

408. Cheng VC, Yew WW, Yuen KY. Molecular diagnostics in tuberculosis. *Eur J Clin Microbiol Infect Dis.* 2005;11:711–720.

409. Sikora M, Interewicz B, Olszewski WL. Contemporary methods for detection of microbial infections in transplanted tissues. *Ann Transplant.* 2005;10:11–16.

410. Mazuchowski EL II, Meier PA. The modern autopsy: what to do if infection is suspected. *Arch Med Res.* 2005;36:713–723.

411. Roberts FJ. Procurement, interpretation, and value of postmortem cultures. *Eur J Clin Microbiol Infect Dis.* 1998;17:821–827.

412. Rosenbloom ST, Stead WW, Denny JC, et al. Generating clinical notes for the electronic health record systems. *Appl Clin Inform.* 2010;1:232–243.

413. Buckley JD, Joyce B, Garcia AJ, Jordan J, Scher E. Linking residency training effectiveness to clinical outcomes: a quality improvement approach. *Jt Comm J Qual Patient Saf.* 2010;36:203–208.

Index